The Doctor Is In

evaluating

Female Hormone Management

The Doctor Is In

evaluating

Female Hormone Management

Audrey L. Ross, N.D.
John F. Whitehorn, M.D., F.A.A.F.P.

One World Press
2000

First Edition published 2000

Library of Congress Control Number: 00-091409
ISBN 0-9644958-4-8

The theories and formulas presented in this book are expressed as the authors' opinions and as such are not meant to be used to diagnose, prescribe, or to administer in any manner to any physical ailments. In any matters related to your health, please contact a qualified, licensed Health Practitioner.

One World Press
P.O. Box 2501
Prescott, AZ 86302
800-250-8171

FOREWORD

As medical professionals the authors have seen great advances involving patients taking a more active roll in their health care decisions. However, disappointments still remain as many allopathic and naturopathic practitioners remain polarized in their treatment decisions, often with limited professional courtesy extended to one another. A main point of emphasis for developing this series of books is to demonstrate the importance of integrating both fields of health care for the benefit of the patient. This integrated approach is highly beneficial to disease prevention, treatment and cure. Education is paramount when making health care decisions and "The Doctor Is In Evaluating..." series of books will provide valuable information regarding both allopathic and naturopathic treatment options.

Dr. John F. Whitehorn is a board certified family practice physician who had the largest singly-physician family practice in Dallas, Texas. He served as Clinical Assistant Professor of Family Practice and Community Medicine at Southwestern Medical School's University of Texas Health Science Center in Dallas. During his 28 year career he was awarded the American Medical Association's "Physician Recognition Award" five times. He also served as President of the Department of Family Practice at Methodist Medical Center in Dallas. He is recognized among his peers for his innovation and development of new treatment modalities. Currently retired from his medical practice, Dr. Whitehorn travels extensively, both nationally and internationally, educating physicians, medical professionals, and lay people about disease prevention, treatment and cure through nutrition, lifestyle choices and stress management.

Dr. Audrey Ross is a practicing Naturopath in Arlington, Texas. After a 17 year career in marketing Dr. Ross returned to school completing her Ph.D. in Naturopathy. As a member of the American Naturopathic Medical Association and the American Nutraceutical Association, Dr. Ross is a highly sought after educational speaker. As a naturopath, natural remedies and treatments are a primary focus, however her understanding of the importance of integrating allopathic practices when necessary sets her apart as a leader in her field.

As supporters of more integrative approaches to treating patients, Dr. Ross and Dr. Whitehorn discovered a common ground, thus beginning a friendship and a professional association representative of the current health care paradigm shift. They have designed this series of books to bring the best of both worlds to the general public and medical professionals. Their effort clearly indicates that allopathic and naturopathic practices can successfully join forces to integrate both medical disciplines to provide the best possible health care options for the patient.

TABLE OF CONTENTS

CHAPTER 1

INTRODUCTION

We are currently facing dramatic changes in our approach to medicine and healing. Natural alternatives are becoming a frequently sought after means of treating illnesses from the common cold to cancer. Unfortunately, our tenacious efforts to identify the correct natural treatment oftentimes result in more confusion and questions than answers. This is why we must step back and realize we need to integrate allopathic (traditional) medicine and naturopathic (natural) healing methods in an effort to provide the most comprehensive form of treatment. The contributions and advances of the modern system of allopathic medicine over the past decades are invaluable, but there is more to learn. Getting back to basics in diet and lifestyle, learning what the alternatives are, understanding natural treatments, and knowing where to go for guidance are all part of regaining optimal health.

This book is the first in a series that will provide understanding to the significance of integrating allopathic and naturopathic practices so that a personal and informed choice can be made about one's health and treatment options. Education is critical in the approach and the decision making process one faces with respect to personal health. The following chapters will provide a resource of necessary and important information that will assist with this process.

First look at what allopathic medicine can and cannot do:[1]

CAN:

- Manage trauma better than any other system of medicine.
- Diagnose and treat many medical and surgical emergencies.
- Treat acute bacterial infections with antibiotics.
- Treat some parasitic and fungal infections.
- Prevent many infectious diseases through immunization.
- Diagnose complex medical problems.
- Replace damaged hips and knees.
- Achieve positive results with cosmetic and reconstructive surgery.
- Diagnose hormonal deficiencies.

CANNOT:

- Treat viral infections.
- *Cure* most chronic degenerative diseases.
- Effectively manage most kinds of mental illness.
- *Cure* most forms of allergy or auto-immune disease.
- Effectively manage psychosomatic illnesses.
- *Cure* most forms of cancer.

---

[1] Andrew Weil, M.D., *Spontaneous Healing,* (New York: The Ballantine Publishing Group, 1995), 225.

Reviewing the list under "cannot," please take special note that *cure* has been used in the categories of chronic degenerative diseases, allergies, auto-immune disease, and cancer. Allopathic medicine can be of great benefit in *treating the symptoms* in these categories, allowing patients the ability to manage the pain and uncomfortable physical affects they experience. However, the body has the natural ability to maintain and heal itself. The individual is responsible for making the choices regarding the type of treatment to undertake, be it allopathic or naturopathic.

It is obvious that people worldwide are focusing on "natural treatments" and are seeking alternative medicine practitioners. However, it is just as important to understand that allopathic medicine should not be completely avoided. It is necessary to focus on integrating the two practices and begin realizing that one can compliment the other, rather than work against one another. In each book of this series the primary goal is to demonstrate that an integrative approach between the two medical practices, for a wide variety of problems, is not only possible but even beneficial to disease treatment and cure.

This book will focus on hormone replacement therapy (HRT) and menopause. This particular topic selection was based on some very specific facts. First and foremost is the reality that there is a great amount of confusion surrounding HRT and menopause. There are conflicting treatment theories, treatment side affects to consider, and, of course, a woman's own physical response. Second, there are almost 33 million women over the age of 65 today. Statistics indicate that every seven minutes another American turns fifty years old. During the next decade the only age group that is expected to experience significant growth is those past the age of 55. By the year 2008 women between the ages of 50 and 65 will be the largest demographic in the nation for the first time in written human history. All of these women will be menopausal! All of them will have questions regarding the best way to get through this "time of change" in their lives.

As the number of women in this age group increases, age related symptoms will arise. We frequently hear the term "mid-life" being used when a woman reports that she "can't remember names anymore," she "feels bloated," she "has no energy," she "has no sex drive," or when someone relates that "she's not herself anymore." We are seeing the impact of this "mid-life market" with the development of age-related product lines as well as voluminous sources of information in print explaining "The Change Of Life" and how to deal with it. Many of these publications are truly worth reading, but other are suspect.

Modern technology has given rise to women's lifestyles and expectations of quality of life that require us to explore those parameters that have the greatest affect in these areas. Traditional medical management of mid-life women must be reassessed, and attention duly given to neuro-hormonal and neuro-chemical activity in response to diet, exercise, stress, toxins and genetic coding. Women are searching for alternatives to traditional medical management of menopause. There is a need to find a way to function without the threat of poorly managed menopause and its potentially harmful consequences. The paradigm shift to natural treatments for other conditions and diseases has motivated women entering menopause to search out knowledge and understanding regarding what is happening to their bodies and how to naturally treat the symptoms associated with hormone fluctuations. Almost daily, new studies are reported about the effects of various hormones, nutritional products and herbs as they relate to the management of mid-life and post-menopausal women. We recognize the value of new ways to treat or prevent these problems, but we must constantly be vigilant not to embrace "treatment fads" and "fountain of youth" drugs. Sensational claims, both positive and negative should evoke suspicion and scrutiny but not necessarily complete rejection. Are all herbs safe? Which ones work best? Should a topical cream be used? What ingredients should be in a topical cream? How is quality control evaluated? Should both herbs and creams be used? The questions are endless! And the answers are even more diverse and far reaching. A progressive and informed approach to mid-life treatments, while subscribing to the time honored treatise of "Do No Harm," is considered the most logical path toward integration of both allopathic and naturopathic healing practices.

Statistics tell us that 15% of women have absolutely no problem with menopause, 15% have severe manifestations, and the rest of the women fall somewhere in between.[2] The hormone roller coaster can begin as early as the age of 35, when many women are at the height of their careers and have enormous family responsibilities. Hormones begin to fluctuate

---

[2] Betty Kamen, Ph.D., *Hormone Replacement Therapy—Yes or No?*,(N0avto: Nutrition Encounter, 1996), 4.

and the annoying side affects begin to occur — depression, bloating, insomnia, irritability, allergies, decreased sex drive, fatigue, foggy thinking, weight gain, water retention, and even hot flashes or night sweats. This is not what the industrialized, professional woman wants to deal with, during what she considers to be the prime of her life! The strong desire to regain control of health issues is what has led women on the search for natural alternatives utilized for the purpose of balancing hormones. But how does one decide what to do?

The numerous conflicting reports add to the confusion. Is it estrogen that is needed to build bones? Why then did the results of a study at the University of British Columbia in Vancouver show a relationship between osteoporosis and progesterone deficiency, not estrogen deficiency? Who do you believe? A major stumbling block women have to face is the conflicting reports and printed material.

Women are entering an age of self-determination and taking on the responsibility of improving their heritage and getting a new lease on life by exerting their power of control. There is an entirely new perspective and approach to menopause today than there was 20 years ago. Today, menopause is considered the antithesis of adolescence. Instead of many hormones raging through the system trying to balance, there are now decreased amounts that are attempting to maintain normal body functions. Hot flashes can be looked at like adolescent acne — an outward sign of a natural process of hormone change that all women go through.[3]

[3] Sadja Greenwood, M.D., *Menopause Naturally: Preparing for the Second Half of Life,* (San Francisco: Volcano Press, 1984), 29.

The information contained in this book will provide very important facts and information needed to make intelligent and informed decisions about the choices one has with regard to hormone replacement therapy. The physical aspects of this aging process are complex and discussed in detail. Some women are very detail oriented and are quite interested in knowing all the statistics and facts regarding the physical transformation the female body encounters. This book will provide all those fine points. For those who have a secondary interest in these details, ***"Speed Notes"*** have been provided throughout the chapters to summarize the main points discussed in each section. However, it is important to have a condensed understanding of what is physically happening to the body to help eliminate some of the fear associated with the unknown. Detail has been included for this reason. The history and physiology of the evolution of menopause will be presented, as well as a brief explanation of the stages women go through during this process.

Information will also be presented regarding prescription hormones and the changes that have occurred over the last several decades. Facts will be supplied to provide a better understanding of the reasons why synthetic hormone use was initiated. Quite often the sensationalism used in reporting problems or side affects overshadow the benefits that some women can get from synthetic treatments. Yes, it is imperative to know all the possible side affects, but it is also important to review this information logically and rationally, keeping the whole picture in perspective. Not every negative reaction will occur. Looking at the pros and cons of prescription hormone replacement therapy needs to be done in conjunction with reviewing all the alternative options and the side affects associated with natural remedies. These options will be discussed in detail.

We must always remember that each woman is an individual and what works for one may not work for another. Studies have shown that in two people there can be a 20-fold difference in blood levels of estrogen with the same prescription oral dose. That is why every woman needs to become more educated with regard to hormone replacement. Learning to interpret the physical symptoms that may be occurring will never be more critical than during menopause. The body knows what it needs and one must simply pay closer attention to the body's signals. Currently there are more physicians at least considering natural hormone replacement options than there were in previous years. What is critical for women to understand is the total effect of synthetic hormones as well as natural remedies. This includes the studies, the findings, the benefits, and the problems.

Although most of the emphasis regarding menopause and hormone replacement revolves around the controversy of synthetic and natural hormones, one very significant topic frequently overlooked is the role of nutrition. The evidence reported clearly indicates that nutrition is a vital key to successfully managing the aging process. As part of the educational information reviewed in this book, nutrition will be thoroughly discussed because of its importance in the equation of menopause management.

There have been more changes in the American diet in the last 50 years than in all of human history. It is essential for women to know how diet, body composition, and exercise can play a dramatic role in making life easier during this mid-life time. Just what really is a "balanced diet"? Is it the same for everyone? What about protein? What about carbohydrates? What about fats? All these questions will be reviewed and discussed providing a better understanding of what has become an increasingly confusing topic. This book will provide an easy to understand guide to nutritional self-management.

It appears that a new diet emerges almost weekly. If any one of these "fads" were truly working for everyone why would there ever need to be a "new" diet program? Frequently clever marketing campaigns and astonishing testimonies will greatly influence perception. Emotions do play a vital role in how one perceives a concept, and when it has to do with health, the emotions run quite high, and perception becomes reality. Compounding this problem during menopause is the fact that fluctuating hormones also affect emotions, thus elevating the potential for perception becoming reality.

Designed to be educational, informative and enriching, the following chapters will provide some basic answers to frequently asked questions regarding the process of aging, known as menopause. Keep in mind, menopause is not a disease! It is a process of aging perhaps best depicted as adolescence in reverse. Our lifestyles have changed dramatically, yet our genetic code is designed for the living conditions of thousands of years ago. The genetic code is the information library in each cell that contains our hereditary information and the functional program for all other cells, tissues and organs. How the body utilizes ingested nutrients as well as the body's reaction to the environment are all part of the genetic code.

As you embark on the educational journey that follows, keep in mind that the purpose of this book is to provide information that will allow you to be able to make intelligent decisions concerning your personal passage through this transitional time of life. All women deserve the opportunity to sort out fact from fiction, and have the choices clearly explained. Integrating both allopathic and naturopathic practices of medicine will allow one to see the whole picture. Confusion, misunderstanding and misdirection permeate the areas of health care and must be approached with caution, yet there must be a willingness to openly evaluate information which will impact each of our lives, as well as the lives of our children.

Learn to enjoy, evaluate and utilize the wisdom and factually based knowledge that will become available. What is done now will impact your quality of life when you are 70, 80 and 90. It is truly a personal choice when it comes to making decisions of what to put in (or on) your body. Shouldn't you have as much information as possible to make these choices? Your journey awaits!

CHAPTER 2

THE EVOLUTION OF WOMEN & MENOPAUSE

The increasing numbers of aging people in the world population have brought changes in the understanding of the biological maturation process including the important role of genetics. Over the past decade insight has been gleaned in areas such as where we came from, how we function and where we are going in our evolutionary process. Genetics has changed the understanding, treatment and prevention of many of the chronic diseases such as arthritis, diabetes mellitus, auto-immune diseases (lupus, fibromyalgia, multiple sclerosis, etc.), neurological diseases, heart disease and cancer, just to name a few. As we begin to understand genetics, it is apparent that a woman's lifestyle must compliment her genetic make-up in order for optimal health to be achieved. The most striking contrast recognized is the lifestyle and longevity of women now as compared to that of thousands of years ago. The body is designed genetically to handle the living conditions and lifestyle that existed thousands of years ago. Human genetic make-up has not changed to accommodate the lifestyle changes of today's living conditions.

DNA

All humans have 23 pairs of genetically laden material called *chromosomes* in each cell of the body. These chromosomes are composed of genes that have special codes (genetic codes) chemically written in DNA. DNA molecules are the basic codes of life that determine sex, skin color, hair color, eye color, etc. More importantly, DNA tells the body how to handle internal biological operation systems such as the depositing of cholesterol in blood vessels, the immune system's response to cancer cells, the ability to build and replace bone, the biological timing of hormone production, the metabolic rate, and much more. These internal biological systems are not easily manipulated, but can be affected by the environment and lifestyle. A question that must be asked is "If human genetic codes are outdated for our current lifestyles, what can be done about it?"

SPEED NOTE

DNA is involved in controlling hormone production, cholesterol levels in the blood, metabolic rate and much more. Lifestyle and environment can positively or negatively affect the proper functioning of DNA.

Lifestyles & Life Expectancies

As recently as 200 years ago, a woman's life expectancy was less than 40 years. The ovaries seldom reached a state of "wearing out" to cause any hormone fluctuations. Also, the lifestyle was certainly much different than today and, the overall body functions, including the endocrine system, were in better operation. As women's life expectancies began to increase, so did the effects of aging. Toward the end of the nineteenth century, the mortality rate for women from childbirth steadily dropped, and diseases began to be more effectively treated. By the year 2050, the life expectancy for women will be almost 85 years. Assuming the average age of menopause is 51 years, women will spend approximately 40% of their life post-menopausal. Menopause is inevitable and represents a substantial portion of a woman's adult life. Quality of life during this period now takes on a new significance! The genetic codes found in modern women with a sedentary lifestyle do not make allowances for this increased life span.

There still are a few native tribes throughout the world who have remained very close to their primitive lifestyles. However, maintaining this native living is becoming more difficult as technology encroaches on these tribes. Historically, tribal women experienced late onset of their menstrual flow, possibly because of the low percentage of body fat. The physical activity these women obtained on a daily basis increased their lean muscles mass and kept the body fat under control. Since body fat is a source of estrogen production, this lower percentage could be the reason why puberty and the onset of menstruation were delayed.

SPEED NOTE

Body fat is a source of estrogen production.

The Menstrual Cycle

The average age of first menstruation was $15\frac{1}{2}$ years. Since the onset of ovulation can occur several years after the first menstruation, childbearing typically did not occur until almost 20 years of age. Then, due to the limited sources of soft foods, women had to breast-feed their children 4-5 years. There were no formal means of birth control and a woman was found to usually have given birth to 4-5 children during her reproductive life. It had been assumed that prehistoric women had given birth to large numbers of children, with most dying in childhood. This is clearly not the case. Because of the prolonged and frequent breast-feeding, women would rarely ovulate. Some investigators believe that breast-feeding prevents the continual exposure to fluctuating higher levels of estrogen that are made in the first part of the menstrual cycle. Without the constant hormone fluctuation the body was able to maintain a better balance and not develop diseases related to excess hormone production.

This is clearly not the standard of modern woman. Today it is not uncommon for a woman to have 400-500 menstrual cycles before menopause. An article in the *Journal of the American Medical Association* discusses "American girls are entering puberty earlier; medical guidelines may need to be changed." The research published attributes this early onset of puberty to diet and environmental factors, such as exposure to external estrogen (xenoestrogen) from hair products, insecticides, and plastics. No modern woman has the lifestyle that mirrors these primitive tribes, nor is that expected to ever recur. What is important is the need to learn what can be done in today's world that will most benefit the health of the female human body.

SPEED NOTE

Early onset of puberty in today's world can be attributed to diet and environmental factors, such as exposure to external estrogen from hair products, insecticides and plastics.

Nutritional Aspects

What can be documented is that when members of these tribes settle into agricultural villages, and forsake their nomadic way of life, changes occur. Instead of forging for nuts, vegetables and wild game, they raise grain and livestock and become sedentary. This results in an increase in overall body weight in addition to an early onset of puberty. Our modern industrialized society has provided a means to improve the quality of life through nutrition, modern medicine and improved sanitation, yet the evolving of the body's genes may never be able to adjust to this new lifestyle.

Modern woman has been provided easy access to food sources, which we know as "fast foods." The majority of these restaurants and retailers serve food that is fried in partially hydrogenated oils and serve items that contain xenoestrogens (to be discussed in detail later). Foods containing fats appeal to our appetite center, which can be partially explained by our genetic code. As nomads, humans did not have the convenience of a grocery store just around the corner to provide a constant food supply. They were subject to the possibility of starvation and thus required high-energy efficient food sources from body storage which we now as fats. These were generally of the polyunsaturated or monounsaturated type and not the saturated variety most commonly found in foods today. These fats, once stored in body tissue, could be used for energy during times when food was scarce. Today, the body still has the craving for fat, but modern society and technology have eliminated the need. One simply needs to get into the car and drive to any number of fast food outlets where that high fat meal will be waiting. Yet even easier, just pick up the telephone and the food will be swiftly delivered, prepared and ready for consumption.

What does all this mean? The DNA inherited from Neolithic ancestors, in most cases, does not allow the body to adequately process the elevated cholesterol and triglycerides found in the typical diet of today. The excess salt frequently found in most foods leaches calcium from the blood and also has a profound negative effect on blood pressure. Both of these conditions, excess calcium loss resulting in osteoporosis and high blood pressure, are two of the symptoms associated with menopause.

SPEED NOTE

Excess dietary salt will leach calcium from the blood as well as increase blood pressure — both symptoms associated with menopause.

Toxins

Further compounding the problem is another set of adaptive stresses for the body to confront. Toxic substances are often difficult to detect and are found in the air we breathe, the water we drink, the food we eat and the physical environment in which we live. Prolonged exposure of the human body to chemicals, both industrial and household, has been shown to disrupt cellular integrity and cause cells to divide and multiply uncontrollably. Cellular integrity is critical during menopause.

Consideration given, the adverse effects on one's health that have been discussed thus far are devastating. Consider the fact that infertility among young couples is constantly increasing and more and more infants are born with birth defects, many not surviving the neonatal stage. Numerous investigators have attributed these findings to toxic substances found in food, water and environment, as well as lifestyle changes. What is being reported in humans can be correlated with a famous study, noted in many books on enzymes and nutrition, involving cats. A 10 year study with 900 cats done by Dr. Francis Pottenger, demonstrated almost the identical reproductive problems caused by improper nutrition. One set of cats was fed raw milk and uncooked meats, while the other set of cats was fed only pasteurized milk and cooked meats or processed foods. The results were remarkable. The cats that ate the raw food were healthy, free of disease and produced healthy offspring for three generations. The cats on the cooked food diet developed allergies, infections and other health problems. As these cats began to reproduce, the second generation had more serious diseases develop and birth defects were more frequent and severe. By the third generation, the cats fed only cooked or processed foods could not even reproduce. This is a very important study that is seldom noted or addressed. Reviewing these results and examining the increase in fertility drugs and clinics, the question that needs to be asked is "Are humans beginning to exhibit health problems equivalent to those noted in this study?"

CHAPTER 3

HORMONES

"It's just her hormones acting up" or "She just needs her hormones adjusted!" How many times have these explanations for a woman's actions been heard? The awareness and affects of hormones is being emphasized in books, newspaper and magazine articles, journals, friends, neighbors, relatives, and even from many doctors. Almost 1.2 million women are entering menopause each year, causing this increased awareness of "hormone replacement," "hormone depletion," "hormone balance" and so on.

Hormone replacement therapy dates back to the early 1950's when hormones were used to treat women whose ovaries were surgically removed.[4] Today it is found that different routes of administration of hormones act to determine their effects on the body. For example, swallowing a tablet containing micronized 17beta-estradiol (Estrace) results in the metalcolic alteration (a bio-transformation) to estrone, which is a weaker metabolite of estradiol. Therefore, it is es-

[4] John R. Lee, M.D., *What Your Doctor May Not Tell You About Menopause,* (New York: Warner Books, 1996), 21.

trone that is markedly elevated in the blood (3-6 times higher) even though 17beta-estradiol was ingested.

Estrogen acts on the liver causing an increased production of heart protective proteins called high-density lipoproteins (HDL) that bind cholesterol while lowering the dangerous low-density lipoproteins (LDL). This is believed to be one of the main reasons that estrogen replacement can help prevent heart disease in post-menopausal women. Oral estrogen has, however, been shown to increase cholesterol in the bile, a condition that predisposes one to gallbladder disease. This is one of the possible adverse side affects of estrogen therapy. The liver also produces two proteins, albumin and globulin, which transport estrogen in the blood to various tissues. The biologically active portion of the hormone (that which acts on tissue) is not attached to these proteins but floats freely in the blood. Therefore, when most blood hormone measurements are taken, the biologically inactive hormone is also measured, thus giving unreliable information about the active hormone level.

What Are Hormones?

Hormones are molecular structures with highly specific spatial configurations and are produced in the body from endocrine glands. They travel throughout the body in the blood stream and act on sensitive tissue sites. Think of a lock and key system with the hormone being a key that can fit into only certain locks, called cell receptors. When a proper fit is found the hormone attaches itself to a receptor on the cell surface enabling the cell to perform a specific function. Estrogen, a sex hormone secreted by the ovary, travels via the blood stream to the uterus where it attaches to certain receptors on cells that result in the growth of uterine lining (endometrium). Other body functions not related to the reproductive system also rely on this same basic mechanism.

Insulin, for example, is a hormone secreted by the pancreas. It attaches to specific receptors on cells resulting in the storage of glucose in the body. Glucose is a basic sugar (carbohydrate) transported in the blood stream which provides an immediate source of energy, such as when you are actively engaged in sports and need the immediate energy. Glucose also serves as the primary fuel for the brain, because of its ability to easily cross from the blood into the nerve cells. Insulin is a good example of how dependent we are on proper hormone secretion and utilization in our everyday activities and existence. If insulin is produced in insufficient quantities, our blood sugar (glucose) can become elevated, which then leads to a condition commonly known as diabetes (mellitus). Without sufficient insulin molecules to act as keys, the cell receptors (or locks) cannot open the needed biological machinery to store excess blood glucose. In certain cases the insulin "key" will not form a proper fit with the cell "lock" and once again, because the biological machinery fails, blood sugar (glucose) becomes elevated. Insulin is included in a group of super-hormones called eicosinoids, which are integrally involved in proper nutrition.

SPEED NOTE

Glucose (blood sugar) provides an immediate source of energy and serves as the primary fuel for the brain. Without sufficient insulin the body cannot store glucose.

It is important to understand the basic concepts of hormone interactions created by an elaborate communication system between the hypothalamus (in the lower portion of the brain), the pituitary gland (at the base of the hypothalamus) and the ovaries (in the pelvis). Each part of this axis communicates with the others via the blood stream to control production of the sex hormones estrogen, progesterone and androgens.

Hormones, receptors and biologic aging are all important in the properly functioning menstrual cycle. The human menstrual cycle is a complex sequence of events that is in a continual dynamic state, the purpose of which is to provide the species the means to perpetuate itself. The hormones that are of importance in this discussion include: 1) estrogen 2) progesterone 3) testosterone 4) follicle stimulating hormone(FSH) 5) luteinizing hormone(LH) and 6) inhibin. Estrogen, progesterone, testosterone (androgen) and inhibin are produced in the ovaries, which form rapidly in embryonic tissue. Genes direct specific tissue in the early stages of development to differentiate into ovaries instead of testes. There are millions of eggs in the ovaries before birth and by puberty, the numbers have decreased to approximately 300,000 in both ovaries. These remaining eggs are located in cell-lined, fluid filled sacs called "follicles." A protective ovarian covering encapsulates the follicles, which themselves are suspended in a supportive structure called "stroma." The stroma is biologically active and is responsible for the production of androgens such as testosterone. Estrogen and progesterone are derived from the cells that line the follicle. Estrogen levels in a normal cycle can be less than 30 pg/ml (a common form of measurement in medicine) in the first few days, but may increase to over 300 pg/ml by the time of ovulation. Progesterone, which first is detected just before ovulation, reaches its highest level about one week after ovulation. The yellowish pigmented corpus luteum, which represents the ovarian follicle left behind after ovulation, produces progesterone. Inhibin is a hormone produced in the follicle, which is important in the modulation of FSH (follicle stimulating hormone).

The Brain & Hormones

The brain is the control center for most of the body's functions. The regions of the brain that are important in the menstrual cycle are the hypothalamus and the pituitary gland. These centers act as conductors in a symphony. They respond to hormonal signals from the ovaries and also from higher brain centers. This simplified model aids in explaining the effects of diet, stress, exercise and other influences on the menstrual cycle. In addition to containing receptors for the ovarian sex hormones, the hypothalamic center also receives input from the neurocortex. After these messages are processed, special signals are then sent from the hypothalamus to the pituitary gland, which secretes two important hormones: FSH (follicle stimulating hormone) and LH (luteinizing hormone). Under the direction of the hypothalamus and the developing ovarian follicle, both FSH and LH travel via the blood to bind ovarian receptors and induce ovarian sex hormone production resulting in ovulation. Production of FSH and LH depends on feedback from estrogen and inhibin. The higher brain centers can also provide feedback in times of emotional stress, sudden weight change and extremely vigorous exercise. These higher brain centers may send messages to the hypothalamic-pituitary system during these times, which can result in hormone imbalances and irregular menstrual cycles. The brain is one of the most sex hormone sensitive organs in the body. While directly orchestrating the menstrual cycle, it simultaneously modulates energy levels, moods, memory, body thermostat and sleep habits using neuro-hormonal connections involving estrogen, progesterone and testosterone.

SPEED NOTE

The higher brain centers can send messages during times of emotional stress, sudden weight changes and extremely vigorous exercise that could result in hormone imbalances and irregular menstrual cycles. The brain also modulates energy levels, moods, memory, body thermostat and sleep habits using estrogen, progesterone and testosterone.

Sex hormones produced under the direction of the pituitary gland travel via the blood to the uterus. The uterus is divided into two basic parts, the muscle layer (myometrium) and the inner layer (endometrium). Nature has also provided the uterus with a generous blood supply assuring adequate nourishment to its cells. The lining continually undergoes changes throughout the cycle. Estrogen is the major stimulus for growth of the uterine lining. Menstrual flow is the shedding of the endometrium indicating that pregnancy did not occur and the hormone levels have declined. The intensity (or heaviness) of the flow is governed in part by the lining thickness. Estrogen provides the initial stimulus for lining growth and in those cycles with excessive estrogen production, heavier flows and large clots are often experienced. Women who begin to have hormonal fluctuation in mid-life may experience shorter and heavier flows. The increase in bleeding reflects the wide swings in estrogen production by the aging ovaries. A marked drop in estrogen production by the ovaries, as seen in menopause, will result in lack of growth of the lining and no menses will occur.

SPEED NOTE

Estrogen provides the initial stimulus for uterine lining growth. Excessive estrogen may result in heavier menstrual flows. A drop in estrogen, as seen in menopause, will result in no menstrual flow.

The lining of the uterus displays a recurring growth pattern in relation to the ovarian hormonal secretion. The first phase (proliferative) is estrogen dominated while the second phase (secretory) includes the addition of progesterone, which acts to further mature the lining. The uterus must be primed hormonally to be able to implant a fertilized egg and nurture a growing embryo into a viable infant. Should pregnancy not occur, the levels of estrogen and progesterone will begin to drop and the uterine lining, deprived of nutrition, will begin to die and slough away (menstruation). The menstrual cycle is dependent on a sensitive hormone feedback system which includes FSH, LH, estrogen, progesterone, and inhibin.

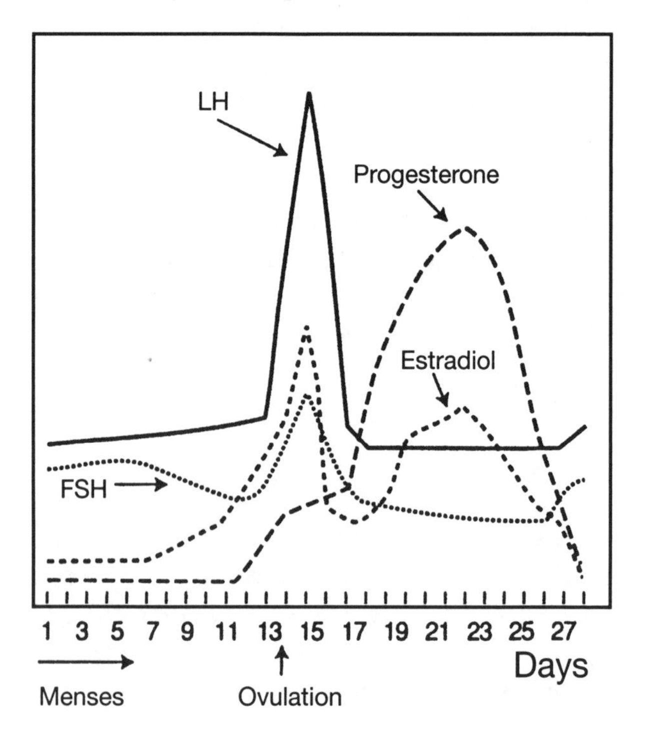

Hormone levels in a normal menstrual cycle.

Estrogen

Estrogen is one of the main hormones produced in the female body. The ovaries, adrenal glands and fatty tissues produce three types of estrogen. 17beta-estradiol is the most potent and plentiful form of estrogen and is primarily produced by the ovarian follicles. Scientists have discovered that the body produces two different types of estradiol: 2-hydroxyestrone, a "good estrogen" that reduces the risk of breast cancer, and 16alpha-hydroxyestrone, a "bad estrogen" that can trigger or stimulate the development of cancer. Estrone is a weaker metaolite of 17beta-estradiol and because this is a reversible reaction, estrone can be converted back to 17beta-estradiol. In post-menopause, the adrenal glands can take androgens and convert them to estrone, which is the predominant estrogen after the onset of menopause. Estriol is the weakest of the natural estrogens and is derived from ovarian estradiol and estrone.

SPEED NOTE

The predominant estrogen after the onset of menopause is estrone, which can be converted from androgens by the adrenal glands.

Estrogen that is derived from outside the body is generally in pill form to be swallowed, in a cream that is applied to the skin (transdermally), injected into the muscle, implanted under the skin, or placed under the tongue (sublingual). 17beta-estradiol, estrone and estriol are available in any of the above forms. Synthetic non-human estrogen derivatives are also used as estrogen substitutes. When referring to estrogen replacement, the term "native hormone" is often used. This refers to a substance synthesized from a source other than the human body, such as Mexican Wild Yam, that has the exact same molecular structure of the human hormone. Estrace is an example of a native hormone replacement. It consists of micronized 17beta-estradiol that has been synthesized from plants but retains the exact chemical structure of the hormone that the ovaries produce. "Native hormones" and "natural hormones" differ only in the place of synthesis.

SPEED NOTE

The term "native hormone" refers to a substance that has the exact molecular structure of the human estrogen produced by the ovaries, but is derived from a source other than the human body. Estrace is an example of a "native hormone."

When Estrace is administered under the tongue, the blood level of estradiol increases rapidly over a few hours. These levels drop within about six hours, which is the reason Estrace should be taken in divided doses in order to maintain its effectiveness. It is not only the *dose* but the *frequency* of taking the hormone that determines its effectiveness.

Transdermal application of estrogen is commonly known as "the patch." Natural estrogen can be placed in a special adhesive matrix that allows a specific rate of hormone release to be absorbed into the blood through the skin, thereby allowing a relatively constant hormone level in the blood. Examples of transdermal preparations are Climara, Vivelle and Estraderm. The type of adhesive and duration of action define each of these products. Since the estrogen is absorbed through the skin it bypasses the liver initially and does not undergo the bio-transformation of oral preparations. Because of this, even though transdermal application creates higher blood levels of estradiol than oral forms, the protective levels of HDL are not increased as much. However, the risk of gallbladder disease is much less.

A gel form of estrogen also exists and can be applied directly to the skin. Estrogen gel, when applied, can be rapidly absorbed into the blood stream in very high concentrations, decreasing over a period of hours and is not sustained as in other delivery forms. Low dose estrogen cream is generally used in the vaginal area to provide high concentration to this sensitive tissue, as well as providing estrogen to the bladder, which is also sensitive to this hormone's stimulation. Gels and creams work especially well for complaints of dryness in the genital area.

Estrogen implants have also been used with success for many years. The pellets are placed below the skin surface in the lower region of the abdomen and generally last for six months. Blood levels are in the upper range of normal and the pellets demonstrate a very even absorption rate into the blood. As with the patch, the hormone implant releases estradiol that does not initially pass through the liver and therefore does not undergo bio-transformation into other metabolites. One advantage with this means of replacement is there is no remembering to take a pill or change a patch.

Contrast this to non-human hormonal estrogen derivatives, which are principally derived from pregnant mares. These derivatives are a mixture of at least nine different conjugated estrogens, which may occur in nature but not in the human body. Premarin [pre (for pregnant)] [mar (for mare)] [in (for urine)] is one of the most common non-human estrogen replacement tablets. These are referred to as "conjugated equine estrogens" (CEE). Native hormonal preparations, such as Estrace, are cleared from the blood stream in hours; Premarin may take weeks. Many of the CEE's are more potent than human 17beta-estradiol and may prevent the body's own 17beta-estradiol from attaching to critical estrogen receptor sites.

SPEED NOTE

Premarin is one of the most common, non-human estrogen replacement tablets, and contains at least nine different estrogens NOT found in the human body.

Another group of non-human hormonal preparations are the Selective Estrogen Receptor Modulators (SERMs). Tamoxifen and Raloxifen are examples of these "anti-estrogens." The term anti-estrogen is not entirely correct since these preparations also exhibit estrogen-like effects. Tamoxifen is used to treat breast cancer survivors with a goal of preventing recurrence.

It is particularly useful against those breast cancers involving estrogen receptors, because Tamoxifen competes with estrogen for the receptor sites. Because Tamoxifen occupies the estrogen receptor site, cancerous cell growth will stop and continued cell division is actually inhibited. Because it exhibits anti-estrogen properties, an intensification of hot flashes, vaginal dryness and sleep disturbances may be noticed. Tamoxifen also exhibits estrogen effects that include preservation of bone mineral density and reduction of death related to heart disease. It can also cause the uterine lining to grow and similar precautions must be followed to prevent uterine cancer, just as if estrogen supplements were being taken. Raloxifen, which inhibits estrogen-sensitive tumor growth, conserves bone mineral density and decreases cholesterol, but unlike Tamoxifen, it does not cause the uterine lining to grow.

SPEED NOTE

Tamoxifen and Raloxifen are two "anti-estrogens" used in treating breast cancer survivors with a goal of preventing recurrence.

Phytoestrogens, estrogen derived from plants, are growing in importance due to research indicating their significance in maintaining health. Phytoestrogens or phytoesterols are structurally and functionally similar to human estradiol. The specific phytoestrogens of interest are "lignans" and "isoflavones," which are 1/400 to 1/1000 as powerful as native estrogens.[5] Lignans are derived from flaxseed, whole grain cereals, vegetables, legumes and fruits. Isoflavones occur in soy, chick peas and some legumes. The role of phytoesterols is believed to be their protective ability to compete for estrogen receptors in the body, thus preventing a continued exposure to high levels of bad estrogen (16alpha-hydroxyestrone). In menopause, and other low estrogen states, phytoestrogens may bind to estrogen receptors and act as replacements for depleted hormones. As an example, plant estrogens, when ingested, may provide certain weak estrogenic effects that act to reduce hot flashes. This could explain why there is no word for "hot flash" in Japan and other countries where phytoestrogens are abundant in the diet.[6] Generous consumption of phytoestrogens, such as soy based products, in the diet may provide supplemental post-menopausal estrogen, which is a form of hormone replacement protecting against osteoporosis and heart disease. Eating 45-50 grams of soy per day would be needed to accomplish this. Additionally, data indicates these plant derived estrogens can act as antioxidants and may lower the risk of cancer, such as breast cancer and colon cancer. The western diet is generally deficient in phytoestrogens when compared to Asian cultures.

---

[5] Betty Kamen, *Hormone Replacement Therapy-Yes or No?*, (Norvato: Nutrition Encounter, 1996), 73.

[6] H.Adlercruetz, et.al., *Dietary Phytoestrogens and the Menopause in Japan*, Lancet 1992: 339; 1233.

SPEED NOTE

Phytoestrogens (plant estrogens) are structurally and functionally similar to human estrogen. Found in soy products, flaxseed, whole grain cereals, fruits, vegetables, legumes, and chick peas, phytoestrogens may act as replacements for depleted hormones. They can also act as antioxidants and may lower the risk of some cancer.

Progesterone

Progesterone is a sex hormone derived mainly from the ovary but is also found in the adrenal glands. Initially, cholesterol is transformed into pregnenolone, which in turn forms progesterone. During the menstrual cycle, progesterone is produced by the ovulating follicle, which becomes the corpus luteum. In this second stage of the cycle, progesterone binds to the receptors in the uterine lining causing a maturing to occur, which serves to prepare the uterus for implantation of the fertilized egg. This is the origin of its name "pro-gestational." This maturing affect is responsible for the prevention of cancer of the uterine lining. While estrogen is responsible for cell division, progesterone is involved with differentiation. Continual exposure of the uterine lining only to the growth stimulating affects of estrogen increases the risk of uterine cancer. Progesterone interrupts this powerful estrogen growth stimulus and thus prevents malignant transformation of the uterine lining.

SPEED NOTE

Progesterone can help prevent uterine cancer.

In addition to progesterone, there are two separate types of synthetic progesterone-like compounds called "progestins" that are used in hormone treatments. A progestin by definition is able to sustain a secretory uterine lining, which occurs in the second part of the menstrual cycle. The available methods for administering progesterone and progestins are not as sophisticated as those related to estrogen delivery. Progestins can be swallowed and subsequently cross the intestines into the blood stream. Provera is one of the most common progestins taken orally. It can be taken once a day since it provides longer sustained blood levels than natural progesterone. Provera can also be given by injection into the muscle in an oil-based form called "Depo-Provera." One injection may last 3-6 months since the hormone is released slowly. Another method of administration is placing capsules containing progestins under the skin. Norplant is an excellent example of this. Progestins, unlike estrogen, do not alter the sex-hormone binding proteins or change blood-clotting factors. They do however have the ability to raise cholesterol levels and decrease the protective HDL in the blood.

Natural progesterone does not pass easily through the intestines, thus must be micronized or in an oil droplet transport system for oral administration. Transdermal routes are a very popular means of delivering natural progesterone. The maximum absorption takes place within 3 hours, then levels decrease over the next 4-6 hours. Natural progesterone does not adversely affect cholesterol levels the way synthetic progestins can. Both natural progesterone and the synthetic progestins can alleviate osteoporosis, but synthetic progestins can result in increased fluid retention, bloating, breast fullness, headaches, and adversely affected moods.

CHAPTER 4

PRE-MENOPAUSE

Approximately 10 to 15 years before the onset of menopause, the ovaries may begin to decrease their production of estrogen, testosterone and progesterone. When a hormone, such as estrogen, drops below a "normal" level in the blood, the brain's neuro-hormonal connections may not function efficiently. Neuro-hormonal connections could best be described as the influence that sex hormones have on the brain's nerves. The critical hormone level required for proper functioning in this area will vary from one woman to another and is unique for each individual. While hormone connections to heart disease and osteoporosis have received a great deal of attention and media coverage, little is mentioned regarding the important neuro-pathways that depend on the daily maintenance of minimum sex hormone levels. The pre-menopause occurs when aging ovaries lead to up and down fluctuations in hormone levels that can lead to acute neuro-hormonal withdrawal symptoms. The most notable symptoms include: 1) fatigue 2) anxiety 3) insomnia 4) headache 5) depression 6) hot flashes 7) mood swings 8) memory lapses 9) "fuzzy" thoughts 10) diminished libido and 11) shorter menses. When a hormone drops below the normal requirement level, the brain does not process its messages in a normal fashion and the subsequent rerouting of the neural signal results in these physical symptoms. The brain is filled with hormone receptors that in turn regulate energy levels, mood, sleep habits, memory and other functions. There are millions of women now entering this phase of life. Some will breeze through without problems, while others will be severely affected by this aging process and will require medical assistance.

SPEED NOTE

Common symptoms of pre-menopause include fatigue, anxiety, insomnia, depression, headache, hot flashes, mood swings, memory lapses, "fuzzy" thoughts, diminished libido and shorter menses.

PMS

An understanding of the interactions of hormones, menstrual cycle and the brain helps guide women through these stressful times. It is important for a health care provider to be attentive and listen to the woman experiencing pre-menopause difficulties. Quite often, the woman's medical history alone will dictate the required treatment. Many of the symptoms may not be consistently present from month-to-month and this tends to confuse the issue. Most women just want to "make sense of what is happening to their bodies."

Women between the age of 35 and menopause tend to have worsening premenstrual syndrome and depression often requiring medical intervention. At some point, usually in the late 30's and early 40's, a woman who is deeply involved in family activities may become dissatisfied with her own life. Subtle changes in her ability to function on a daily basis are worrisome and frustrating; memory can become a problem and recollection of words difficult. At home there may be a lack of energy, increased family disharmony, and irregular menstrual cycles. Early morning headaches are not relieved by medicine cabinet analgesics. Awakening in the middle of the night in a drenching sweat and insomnia become tiring and commonplace. *Down* days outnumber the *up* days especially the week before the menstrual flow. Hands swell to the point of preventing the removal of rings and one begins to wonder if this is the beginning of menopause. At this point, a vicious cycle may develop because the more medical care is sought, the more one is labeled hysterical, causing life to become truly miserable with little hope to make it better. Attempts to get medical help quite often result in being given antidepressants, sleeping pills or vitamins. Not only do these things not work but, they may actually make the individual feel worse after using them. Routine hormone lab tests performed at the doctor's office may be completely normal; therefore, menopause is not diagnosed and hormone replacement is not considered the answer.

Hormone Functions

Insufficient hormones, especially estrogen, may be responsible for many of the devastating pre-menopausal symptoms. It should be emphasized that because of the continual monthly fluctuation of ovarian hormones, laboratory testing in not always helpful in diagnosis. As a result of unremarkable lab values and the lack of understanding neuro-hormonal connections, many women are denied proper medical advice from health care professionals.

The female brain is awash in a hormonal milieu of estrogen, progesterone and androgen-like substances such as testosterone. Although the benefits of estrogen have been touted, it is now apparent that the neuro-hormonal connections influencing the microcircuits in the brain are of extreme importance. Think of the brain as a personal computer that consists of billions of biologic microcircuits, which form telecommunication highways that interconnect both its storage and communications centers. Messages are transmitted in the brain along the circuit highways by nerves in the form of electrical impulses that in turn release small packages of powerful chemicals called "neurotransmitters." The neurotransmitters are the nerve's original electric signal now converted into a chemical message that is being passed on to other parts of the brain's control center. Ultimately, the brain's intercommunication, information gathering and final output depend on both electrical and chemical packages. This is a biological internet being composed of multiple chemical switchboards. Messages that travel down these microcircuits help the brain control body temperature, sleep, emotions, memory and moods. The most glaring oversight is the multiplicity of influences on this delicate system. Hormones, foods consumed, ingested and non-ingested chemicals, water, exercise levels and other lifestyle habits are only a few of the elements that can influence this "neuro-net."

Why is estrogen so important? At the microscopic level, estrogen increases the surface area and the number of nerve branchings, therefore allowing more exchange of information with other nearby brain centers. In the laboratory, estrogen has induced nerves to grow within 5 minutes of exposure. Inadequate estrogen levels would result in decreases in nerve growth factors called "neurotrophins" and brain derived growth factor in the cerebral cortex and hippocampus, both estrogen sensitive regions in the brain. The cerebral cortex, which contains many estrogen receptors, acts to process neuro-net signals that control abstract reasoning, planning, language, sensory perception and long term memory storage. The hippocampus is involved in short term information processing and storage. These are but a few examples of how optimal estrogen levels work with the brain's microcircuitry to promote improved cognition, mood stabilization and enhanced mental performance. Hence, estrogen plays an important role in both short and long term memory. The inability to recall a friend's name or having difficulty arranging numbers can be related to estrogen sensitive functions of the brain.

Although the exact mechanism is not fully understood, it is known that estrogen increases blood flow to the brain while stimulating the growth of critical nerve endings and the production of various neurotransmitters such as serotonin. Some antidepressants, such as Prozac, act by maintaining serotonin levels in the brain. Mid-life is when women frequently exhibit more depression and anxiety than their male counterparts, with this difference disappearing in the post- menopausal years. Without clear cut lab values to indicate menopause, physicians will often resort to using antidepressants when other methods of health care, such as dietary changes and exercise, are more appropriate. Certainly, all depression is not hormonally derived, but a careful and in depth interview with the female patient will assist in formulation of an appropriate treatment plan.

Estrogen is also responsible for the secretion of natural mood elevators called "endorphins." These act as natural opiates and are increased by exercising, which is the basis of what have been termed "the runners' high." One of the possible long-term effects of estrogen is the protection against the onset of Alzheimer's disease. Ongoing clinical trials are underway, the results of which may establish a positive beneficial role of estrogen as it relates to Alzheimer's disease.

SPEED NOTE

Estrogen may protect against the onset of Alzheimer's disease. Estrogen also is responsible for the production of endorphins — natural mood elevators.

As estrogen levels begin to decline, neurocircuits regulating the brain's thermostat being to malfunction, resulting in "hot flashes." It is of little wonder that since these can occur at night, sleep patterns can be interrupted resulting in insomnia. Lack of uninterrupted sleep leads to daytime irritability, which becomes a problem for today's woman whose responsibilities do not permit taking time off to rest and catch up on lost sleep. Sleep deprivation, hot flashes, declining levels of natural mood elevators and natural antidepressants certainly explain why the woman may exclaim "I sometimes just cry, and cry for no reason at all!"

Headaches

Headaches are a major health concern for premenopausal women and are experienced at least three times more frequently than in men. Gender differences regarding headaches appear at the onset of puberty and begin to subside at post-menopause. Approximately 95% of headaches are either migraine or tension related. Characteristics of a menstrual migraine are: 1) throbbing pain on one side of the head 2) rarely heralded by an aura 3) accompanied by nausea and vomiting 4) sensitivity to light and sound 5) duration from 4 to 24 hours and 6) triggered by decreased levels of estrogen. At least 40% of women notice an increase in headaches during pre-menopause, the severity of which may require bed rest or even medical assistance. The headaches usually begin several days prior to menses and may extend up to 5 days into the flow, with most disappearing before the menstrual flow has stopped. Some women report an increase in headaches during the second half of the cycle, in conjunction with PMS, while others report occurrence at mid-cycle. The role of estrogen in the menstrual migraine may best be explained by the knowledge that estrogen is a vasodilator (dilates blood vessels in the brain) and estrogen is responsible for increased production of serotonin in the brain. Serotonin attaches to certain receptors in the brain that reduce pain from migraines.

Other causes of hormonal headaches can be attributed to the fact that as the lining of the uterus begins to break down at the time of menses, it releases substances called prostaglandin. Current medications such as ibuprofen, block prostaglandin formation. Although a hormonal relationship is certainly present, causal agents such as stress, certain foods and barometric pressure can also trigger headaches. A thorough review of all causal agents should be completed to determine the proper course of treatment.

Other Symptoms & Causes

Pre-menopausal uterine bleeding is another troubling and unpredictable symptom. The pre-menopausal woman is more likely to have structural abnormalities such as uterine fibroids, which can cause heavy flow during menstruation. The menstrual cycle may be shortened from the normal 28 days to 21 days because of the rapid follicle growth from elevated FSH. Overcompensation by the ovaries can lead to "estrogen dominance," producing symptoms of bloating, breast tenderness and agitation. Chapter 3 discusses the hormone process during a menstrual cycle.

Months of decreased estrogen production will be characterized by spotting or light menstrual flow. When low estrogen levels occur, especially in the second part of the cycle, worsening of premenstrual symptoms (PMS) may be experienced. The excess progesterone in relation to the lower estrogen may block estrogen receptor functions. A lower than normal estrogen to progesterone ratio indicates that the estrogen has dropped below its critical level, consequently, PMS symptoms such as mood swings, sweet cravings, bloating, headaches, insomnia, anxiety and fatigue may be experienced. These tend to occur approximately two weeks before the menstrual flow begins.

After ovulation has occurred, progesterone is made by the ovary. As the pre-menopausal ovaries age, the production of progesterone can be insufficient or short-lived. The lack of adequate progesterone may be reflected by a shortened menstrual cycle or, in some cases, the worsening of PMS. Progesterone is nature's anti-anxiety hormone and has a calming affect while also serving to decrease breast tenderness and bloating.

The majority of women suffering from severe PMS seem to be estrogen deficient as opposed to progesterone deficient, therefore, we treat the second part of the menstrual cycle with natural estrogen supplements initially but may switch to natural progesterone if needed. The main culprit in pre-menopause is the fluctuation of estrogen below the body's normal levels with subsequent neuro-hormonal abnormalities. When the ovary does not release an egg (anovulatory cycle), there is no production of progesterone and subsequent delays in menstrual bleeding may ensue. These delays may range up to several months and can be followed by heavy flows. Anovulatory cycles seem to be well tolerated since estrogen is not fluctuating as in the normal menstrual cycle. These prolonged cycles may be experienced on occasion but as the ovary is depleted of healthy follicles, the cycles become more frequent and finally cease, resulting in menopause.

SPEED NOTE

The majority of women suffering from severe PMS seem to be estrogen deficient rather than progesterone deficient.

Women who suffer from the symptoms believed to be pre-menopausal should carefully select a health care provider who will take adequate time to listen and evaluate all symptoms. Listening to the patient is a key element in pre-menopausal treatment. Following the initial visit to the well trained health care provider, and using the information gathered in this evaluation, a multifaceted treatment plan is tailored using 1) natural hormone replacement 2) nutrition 3) mental wellness and 4) gynecologic wellness. The more devastating pre-menopausal symptoms such as depression, fuzzy memory, fatigue, insomnia, headaches and anxiety may have neuro-hormonal connections, and will respond well to hormone replacement therapy. It is best to begin with a low dose natural estrogen preparation containing 17beta-estradiol. These natural hormones are plant-derived and bio-identical, having the identical molecular structure, as the hormones the body produces. Natural preparations seem to act as better keys to fit into the body's hormonal receptor locks. Fewer side affects are observed with these plant-based hormones than with the non-human synthetic brands. Symptoms improve within days to weeks. A specific replacement regimen must be designed for each woman.

SPEED NOTE

Because of the identical molecular structure of natural plant-based hormones, fewer side affects are observed than with non-human synthetic brands.

If a uterus is present, natural progesterone is added to the estrogen supplementation regimen to prevent the over-stimulation of the uterine lining with estrogen. Synthetic progestins should be avoided because of the unacceptable side affects. Natural progesterone has a place in the treatment of PMS symptoms and has fewer side affects than synthetics such as Provera or Aygestin. Progesterone *de-excites* in contrast to estrogen, which *excites*.

Means of monitoring treatment include observing blood estrogen levels and periodic transvaginal sonography (to monitor uterine lining thickness and consistency). Using this technology, painful endometrial biopsy is rarely needed.

Vaginal dryness, another pre-menopausal symptom, can result in painful intercourse, but can be successfully treated with a natural estrogen gel applied directly to the vagina. Estradiol and estriol gels are both available, with estriol the weakest of the body's natural estrogens. Estriol does not cause breast tenderness and causes very little growth of the uterine lining. Bladder problems, including loss of urine or the urge to urinate frequently, can also be experienced in the pre-menopausal years. These may be the results from lack of estrogen and a similar treatment program may be instituted. Estradiol and estriol may be used in combination to avoid the swelling, bloating and breast tenderness associated with excessive amounts of estrogen.

Hormone Replacement Cautions

Contraindications to estrogen replacement therapy include: 1) abnormal liver function 2) active gallbladder disease 3) acute blood-clotting problems 4) elevated triglycerides 5) pulmonary embolism 6) vascular stroke 7) unexplained uterine bleeding 8) pregnancy and 9) estrogen sensitive cancers.

Exclusive use of natural hormones is preferable; however, the need for contraception in the pre-menopausal woman should not be overlooked. The unplanned pregnancy rate for women in their forties is comparable to that of their teenage counterparts. In certain cases, if contraception is needed in addition to estrogen replacement, low dose estrogen dominant birth control pills with weak progestin effects can be used, such as Ovcon-35 and Ortho tri-cyclen.

Contraindications to taking oral contraceptives in the pre-menopausal years include the same contraindications to natural estrogen replacement plus 1) smoking 2) elevated serum cholesterol and triglycerides 3) the presence of migraines that are heralded by aura and 4) a strong family history of heart disease. Pre-menopausal women may use oral contraceptive pills up to the age of 50.

SPEED NOTE

The unplanned pregnancy rate for women in their forties is comparable to that of their teenage counterparts. Pre-menopausal women may use birth control pills up to the age of 50.

Testosterone

The pre-menopausal ovary can also decrease its production of androgens such as testosterone, causing symptoms such as 1) a decrease in sense of well being 2) a decrease in aggressive energy 3) a decrease in libido and 4) a decreased sensitivity in the clitoris. Testosterone is not just a male hormone and should not be overlooked in hormone replacement therapy. Like estrogen treatment, natural testosterone replacement is not only dependent on laboratory values but also on symptom analysis. Supplementation with natural testosterone preparations should be considered in the pre-menopausal woman experiencing any of the above symptoms and with lower than normal lab values of testosterone. Using low doses will prevent unwanted side affects such as increased facial hair growth, oily skin or voice changes. It is extremely unfortunate that testosterone replacement is associated with these undesirable changes. Many women who could have benefited from replacement have either been denied treatment or have been needlessly alarmed by erroneous information. Most of the adverse side affects have occurred with very large doses of synthetic testosterone.

Administration of testosterone can be either transdermally or sublingually. The transdermal cream is very soothing and is generally applied to the back of the hands, abdomen, inner thighs or vulvar region on a rotational basis. Blood levels of testosterone are monitored to ensure proper dosing. Because of the increased surge of energy, it is not wise to take testosterone late in the day since insomnia may occur. By taking testosterone in the morning women can experience that surge of energy for the remainder of the day. Maximum relief of symptoms may not be experienced for up to five weeks because testosterone must travel into the cell nucleus and begin to rebuild needed proteins, a process that requires time.

SPEED NOTE

Testosterone is often overlooked in pre-menopause treatment because of sensationalized reports of adverse side affects. Many women can benefit from low dose testosterone supplementation during pre-menopause.

Thyroid gland malfunction can cause similar symptoms as those found in estrogen deficiencies. Women have a higher incidence of thyroid abnormalities than men have. Thyroid gland function is easily assessed by blood tests and should be incorporated in the pre-menopausal woman's evaluation.

The Vital Role Of Nutrition

This discussion would be far from complete if proper nutrition were not included. In order to obtain maximum benefit from the natural hormonal replacement recommendations that are presented, one must undertake a healthy lifestyle that would include proper nutrition and adequate exercise. Chapter 6 of this book goes into great detail and explanation about the importance of food, the foods to eat, the foods to avoid, and the importance of a healthy lifestyle. Chapter 6 should be read and studied to provide the education needed to maximize the benefits of natural hormone replacement therapy.

Food is one of the most important drugs that can be ingested on a daily basis and therefore should be treated as such. Beware of the high glycemic, high carbohydrate foods that cause elevated blood insulin levels followed by extreme fatigue several hours later. Most people have experienced the heavy carbohydrate noon meal and the subsequent yawning and sluggishness for the rest of the afternoon. Eat meals every 4-5 hours consisting of 40-60% carbohydrates, 20-30% protein and a **maximum** of 20% fat. A personal caloric intake is determined by the amount of exercise completed each day. Good nutrition includes adequate amounts (70-80 ounces) of chemical free water, 20-30 grams of fiber each day, essential fats (from fish, soy, olives, avocados and nuts) and 5-9 servings of fresh raw fruits and vegetables. Basic nutritional considerations should include all of these. Refer to Chapter 6 to ascertain the details.

Other nutritional suggestions would include:

- Use mostly low glycemic foods. (refer to chart in Chapter 6)

- Steam, bake or even microwave foods — avoid charcoal cooking or frying.
- Use foods that are NOT processed, since processing generally removes many nutrients.
- Avoid adding salt.
- Minimize canned food use, especially if PMS is a problem.
- Refrain from eating foods with refined sugars, like candy.
- Include garlic, preferably fresh, in food preparation.
- Avoid caffeine.
- Limit alcohol.
- Stop smoking.
- Increase consumption of "phytoestrogens" from soy products, papayas, flax and whole grain products.

Exercise

Exercise cannot be emphasized enough in the premenopause phase of life, especially for maintaining weight, enhancing mental well being, strengthening bones and providing cardiovascular protection. Due to distractions such as television and our increased mechanized society, most everyone falls far short of the needed activity required by the body. As the body's metabolic rate declines with age, physical activity becomes much more important in maintaining proper body weight. It is wise to avoid a diet program that does not include a designed exercise plan. Exercise releases "endorphins" that are natural mood enhancers. These substances become very important in warding off depressive states and helping deal with stress. Daily exercise is especially useful for mood enhancement during the second half of the menstrual cycle when PMS can become disabling.

Osteoporosis & Heart Disease

It is important to think long term with regard to osteoporosis and heart disease. Weight bearing exercise strengthens bone and prevents its breakdown. Many women in the pre-menopausal years already have osteoporotic bone changes that can worsen in the post-menopausal years unless corrective steps are undertaken now. Exercise routines should be designed to burn fat and increase or maintain cardiovascular and respiratory fitness. An aerobic exercise regimen that stresses prolonged fat burning exercises such as brisk walking for 45-60 minute periods, at least 5 times per week, is recommended. The intensity of the exercise should be dictated by the heart rate, the number of heart beats per minute. A guide to figure target heart rate would be as follows:

(220 - your age) x 70% =
target heart rate for fat burning

Therefore, for a 45 year old the target heart rate would be 122, based on the calculation (220 - 45) x 70% = 122. This is only a guide and it is always recommended to check with a qualified health care provider before beginning any diet or exercise program. The goal of an exercise program is to lower blood pressure, maintain proper levels of blood lipids (fats), strengthen the heart muscle and decrease its workload through weight control.

SPEED NOTE

Exercise is important in maintaining body weight, cardiovascular health and bone density. Both aerobic and weight bearing exercise are important.

Stress

Stress is ever present and proper management of stress must be considered in every long-term treatment plan. Although stress is not limited to pre-menopause, it does seem to be overwhelming at that time because of the fluctuations of hormones that disturb the neuro-hormonal balance. Financial problems, job dissatisfaction and family difficulties seem to be the most common reasons for stress in modern society. Maintaining acceptable life styles have forced many women into the job market and caused them to abandon their traditional role in the family unit, often times requiring long hours of work at the office. Attempting to run a home, which may include caring for children, a husband and/or aging parents, while maintaining a job is extremely demanding and can lead to considerable stress. Most often, the woman neglects her own health, both physically and mentally, which then leads to a breakdown of systems. When this happens, and the body's coping mechanisms begin to falter under the intense stress, a woman may complain of severe PMS, anxiety, depression, fatigue, decreased libido, headaches, irritable bowel syndrome and the list continues.

Many sources dealing with stress reduction suggest focused breathing exercises that involve self-meditation. Unfortunately, western medicine has neither adopted nor emphasized the power of "mind over body" and instead substitutes pills in place of relaxation techniques. One can be rather creative in finding ways to mentally relax. In addition to breathing or physical exercise, try listening to soothing music or view pleasant scenery such as art or floral arrangements. Consider taking a 24 hour "news fast" during which you neither listen to nor read about the world's insanity. Although nutrition, exercise and stress reduction are important, other treatment options may still be required.

Antidepressants

There are some instances where the previously discussed treatments do not have significant affects. Use of antidepressant medications such as seretonin re-uptake inhibitors (Zoloft, Paxil, Prozac or Serazone) should be reserved for those women with moderate depression requiring more than conventional treatment. This form of treatment should be limited to less than six months duration, which allows for resolution of the stress producing events. Ultimately the problem(s) must be faced and resolved.

Gynecologic Health

The functional well being of the internal organs assumes great importance in the pre-menopause years. Common complaints of a physical nature during this time include 1) increased menstrual flow 2) irregular flow patterns 3) pelvic pain 4) loss of bladder control 5) prolapse of the vagina or uterus 6) bowel difficulties and 7) ovarian or uterine masses. Today's gynecologist has the advantage of sophisticated technology, which was not available in the recent past. The above noted gynecological problems can be readily treated by a competent physician.

With over 20 million women entering the pre-menopausal phase of life, many will experience neuro-hormonal symptoms that can be quite debilitating. When medical advice is sought, many will be denied hormonal treatment based on the results of laboratory values indicating a non-menopausal state. Pre-menopause symptoms should be the guide for natural hormone replacement. Even though menstrual flows are still present, the brain may be suffering from lack of hormones, especially estrogen. A complete evaluation, which should include a discussion of what is happening to the body. A physical exam and appropriate laboratory studies act as guides for the personalization of the treatment plan. When hormone treatment is indicated, only natural hormonal preparations should be employed. A healthy lifestyle must compliment hormonal therapy in order to achieve optimal wellness. Lifestyle encompasses nutrition, exercise, stress reduction and gynecological wellness. The motivation to comply with a medically sound treatment plan can help negotiate the hormonally turbulent pre-menopause time and maintain optimal health through the post-menopausal years.

CHAPTER 5

MENOPAUSE

Many women welcome menopause and view it as the time of rest and solitude after the tumultuous pre-menopause. For many women menopause means the ovaries no longer have any eggs, therefore, sex hormones such as estrogen are no longer produced. Others view it as a mythical point in life where the effects of aging suddenly become more pronounced. At the end of the 19th century, the average woman's life expectancy coincided with the age of menopause. Now that life expectancy can be extended into the eighties, the increasing number of women entering into this phase of life has pressured modern medicine to provide a means to maintain optimal health and wellness. Menopause may occur through natural means or result artificially through surgery. Natural menopause, which we hold to be synonymous with a gradual decrease in the production of ovarian sex hormones over a period of years, is really a retrospective diagnosis and somewhat imprecise. A woman must have no menses for a period of 12 months due to permanent loss of ovarian function to be considered to be in menopause. Other conditions such as polycystic ovaries, pregnancy, chemotherapy, radiation, leukemia or other cancers can cause ovarian failure and must be excluded. Blood tests measuring FSH and estrogen may be used as final confirmation of menopause. Hot flashes and other menopausal symptoms may be experienced before actual menopause is reached. The average age of natural menopause is between 50.5 and 51.5 years of age. Almost 95 of women will be menopausal between the ages of 45 and 55, while only 5% will reach this stage before the age of 45. Humans are unique in that other mammals generally do not live beyond their reproductive years, whereas human menopause simply signals the end of reproductive capability. With a life span of almost 85 years, a woman may spend 40% of her life post-menopausal. Natural menopause is preceeded by the gradual decline in ovarian hormone production, which has been reviewed in the pre-menopausal discussion in Chapter 4. Natural menopause begins years before the final menstrual flow and the symptoms will not always be the same as those experienced in artificially induced (such as surgical) menopause.

SPEED NOTE

The average age of natural menopause is between 50.5 and 51.5 years old.

Pre-menopause, peri-menopause and climacteric are examples of names that have been used to describe the phases a woman goes through before experiencing complete ovarian failure. The terms pre-menopause and climacteric have been used to describe women from their mid-thirties onward who begin to notice symptoms attributed to a decrease in ovarian hormone production, including estrogen, progesterone and even testosterone. The term peri-menopause refers to the time immediately before and after menopause. As menopause approaches, menstrual cycles become further apart and finally stop altogether.

Hormones & Menopause

The primary etiology (cause) of "natural" menopause is the declining number of hormone producing follicles in the ovary. With approximately 1 million follicles at birth, this number decreases to about 300,000 at puberty, 40,000 at 35 years of age, and very few to zero after menopause. The follicle is the primary production site for both estrogen and progesterone. The estrogen that is found at menopause is primarily that which is produced by fat cells converting androgenic hormones to "estrone." Estrone is one of the three natural estrogens. With the ovary losing follicles and decreasing its production of estrogen, the brain responds by increasing the secretion of FSH (follicle stimulating hormone), which is designed to stimulate the ovarian follicles. In addition to the increased release of FSH, LH (leutinzing hormone) is also released in greater quantities. Even though the menopausal ovary, for all intents and purposes, has ceased production of estrogen and progesterone, it is far from being dormant hormonally. The ovarian connective tissue (stroma) that once supported follicles is alive with hormone production. This matrix of tissue, which forms the body of the ovary, gives rise to testosterone. This tissue is sensitive to LH which increases post-menopausally and in turn stimulates the stroma to secrete greater levels of testosterone and other androgenic hormones. Fat cells can then convert these androgens to estrone.

SPEED NOTE

Fat cells can convert testosterone and other androgen type hormones to the natural estrogen known as estrone.

Menopause Hormones

Androgens are manufactured not only by the ovary but also by the adrenal glands, located on top of the kidneys. Three androgens that are especially important are testosterone, DHEA (dehydroepiandrosterone) and androstenedione. "Andros" means male-like, and herein lies one of the misconceptions that "androgens are not that important in women but only in men." Doctors and women alike associate the affects of androgen replacement with the side affects of increased hair growth (especially facial hair), acne, deepened voice and even increased muscle size. These are not seen with normal dosage; however, the masculine side affects occur primarily when large pharmacologic doses of synthetic androgens are administered. In fact, normal blood levels for a woman can be achieved using natural testosterone preparations and this can relieve many pre- and post-menopausal difficulties. Androstenedione and DHEA are secreted by the ovary in greater quantities than is testosterone. Cholesterol is metabolized to pregnenolone, which is then converted to DHEA, which in turn is converted to androstenedione. Testosterone is subsequently derived from the conversion of androstenedione and androstenediol. Estradiol is then derived from the bio-transformation of testosterone. These reactions can be thought of as having a cascade-like affect, which results in the primary production of estrogen using androgen hormones. Some of the androgens are diverted to form estrogen and others form testosterone. DHEA and androstenedione have very low biologic activity and are not potent androgens, but they can serve to form a hormonal reservoir from which the body can metabolize other necessary active hormones as just described. Testosterone, one of these active hormones, is the most powerful circulating androgen in a woman. During reproductive years, the ovaries account for 25% of the total testosterone production and 50% of all androstenedione production. The ovary is a major manufacturer of androgens.

SPEED NOTE

Testosterone and other androgens are used to form estrogen in the menopausal woman. Testosterone is the most powerful androgen in a woman. Small doses of natural testosterone can relieve many pre- and post-menopausal difficulties.

The adrenal glands are another source of androgen production, and in the reproductive years, the adrenal glands produce almost 90% of the total DHEA and 100% of DHEAS, which is the metabolic form of DHEA. Almost all DHEA is rapidly converted in the body to DHEAS. The adrenal glands are responsible for almost 50% of the androstenedione and 25% of the testosterone in the blood.

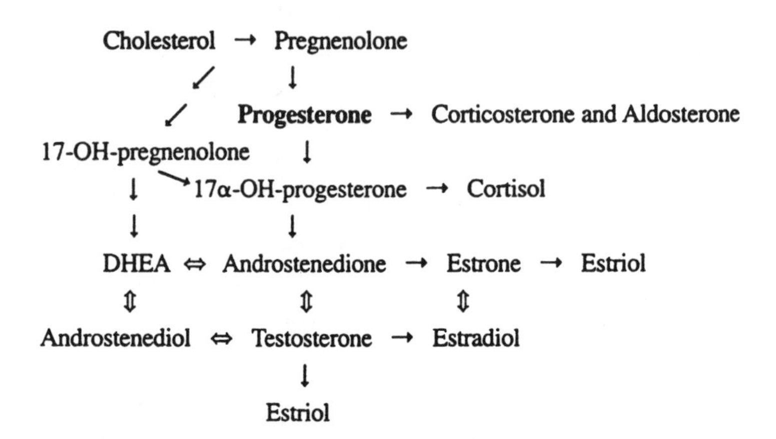

The onset of menopause not only brings about changes in the ovaries but also in the adrenal glands. This "adrenopause," as it is sometimes labeled, is hastened by menopause. There appears to be a common link because the decreased hormonal production of the ovary is also accompanied by a decrease in adrenal gland activity. The follicles in the ovary may no longer function in the post-menopausal state, but the ovarian connective tissue (stroma) still responds to the stimulatory effects of brain derived hormones such as FSH. This stroma response is seen in the increased production of testosterone and androstenedione. Almost 50% of the post-menopausal woman's testosterone is derived from ovarian sources, even though the overall menopause androgen level is still decreased.

At age 40, androgen levels are approximately 50% of the levels at age 20. Decreased adrenal function may be responsible for this change.

Another indication of adrenal slow down is seen in the age-related decline in levels of DHEA. DHEA is derived from pregnenolone almost entirely in the adrenal glands. The levels peak in the third decade of life and then begin to decline. This decline can be linked to a decrease in testosterone levels. Even though the ovarian stromal component may increase androgen production, a decline in adrenal function leads to lower overall androgen levels. This may account for the increase in symptoms seen in menopause.

Testosterone

Attention should be turned to testosterone, being the most powerful androgen in a woman's body. It is indeed unfortunate that more attention has been given to the rarely occurring masculinizing affects of this hormone than to its important roll in day-to-day existence. Men tend to produce almost 20 times more testosterone than women but still the female hormone tapestry would not be complete without it. Testosterone deficiency has been associated with 1) loss of libido 2) decreased feeling of well being 3) decreased energy 4) difficulty reaching orgasm 5) thinning and loss of hair in the genital area 6) scalp hair breaking more easily 7) skin dryness 8) decreased sensation in the clitoris and breast nipples and 9) genital atrophy. These symptoms frequently occur, but in many cases the cause is not investigated and the symptoms are left untreated.

Testosterone can promote an active outgoing self-assertiveness in a woman that may be of particular importance in a "male dominated business world." For those women who are business professionals, success often depends on their ability to be assertive, aggressive and self confident. Some studies have actually shown higher levels of testosterone in these highly motivated women.

In addition to mood and energy changes, testosterone can increase libido, frequency of sexual fantasies, the urge to masturbate and heighten the erotic sensitivity of both the clitoris and breast. The brain's sexual energy is very dependent on the amount of testosterone present. Recent studies indicate that testosterone is implicated in the building of strong bone. It is interesting to note that testosterone alone does not seem to prevent osteoporosis but works in combination with estrogen to actually help the body make new bone.

Almost 10 years prior to the onset of natural menopause androgens, including testosterone, begin to slowly decline. This insidious decline may not be dramatic enough to produce symptoms immediately. A careful history of symptoms is required to determine if testosterone replacement is needed. Simply measuring the amount of testosterone in the blood will not give an accurate assessment of hormonal needs. This is because testosterone is attached to a protein called "sex hormone binding globulin" or SHBG, which circulates in the blood. Since SHBG is protein bound, it cannot bind with the cell receptors and is biologically inactive (useless). The active and important state is in a much smaller quantity. Free testosterone can bind with the cell receptors and initiate cell reaction.

Anything that tends to increase SHBG will decrease the free testosterone and lower its biologic activity. Estrogen increases SHBG, thus estrogen replacement can in fact lower needed testosterone levels. Conversely, obesity tends to lower SHBG and more testosterone is freed from its bound inactive state. Obesity may then provide more free testosterone for the body to use.

How is the need for testosterone supplementation determined? One of the most important components in this determination is that the health care provider needs to listen carefully to the patient. If the patient manifests any of the symptoms previously noted, testosterone supplementation may be required and a health care provider with hormonal expertise should be consulted. The accurate identification of a woman's symptoms is just as important as the results of her blood tests. Hormonal blood evaluations should be taken during the first part of the menstrual cycle, generally around day 3, with day 1 being the first day of normal flow. It is at this time that hormone levels are at base levels. Women should be considered for testosterone treatment when they have significant symptoms and total testosterone levels are low. It cannot be overemphasized that one should not be treated solely on the basis of laboratory test results.

Surgical Menopause

In the United States, one of the most common surgical procedures for women between the ages of 30 and 54 is the hysterectomy. The term hysterectomy implies the removal of the uterus. Annually, 100,000 of these operations will also include removal of the ovaries. Surgical menopause occurs when women have their ovaries removed prior to the natural event of menopause. These women experience acute hormonal deficiencies that can result in a 50% drop in the body's testosterone levels within 24 to 48 hours of the operation. Needless to say this is a severe shock to the system since the brain and body have virtually no time to acclimate. Because of the lack of hormones, the testosterone receptors on the cell will be empty and will result in improper neural signals to the brain or inappropriate cell reactions. Natural menopause is a gradual decrease in hormone levels that permits time for the body to adjust. In surgical menopause, not only is there a sudden decrease in the levels of sex hormones such as testosterone, but also the ovarian hormones. Some suggest that pre-operative measurements of testosterone should be taken to ensure proper and adequate post-operative dosing. The post-operative healing process is also hastened by testosterone.

Testosterone Supplementation

Once the need for testosterone has been determined, the proper course of supplementation must chosen. Prior to the actual administering of testosterone, adequate estrogen must first be replaced since estrogen can increase the number of testosterone receptors on the cell. It may take several weeks to appreciate full affects because the necessary cellular machinery must first be restored. If acne or excessive body hair growth has been a problem, testosterone supplementation should be carefully evaluated. New outbreaks of acne are infrequent but can occur. Increased body or facial hair and deepening of the voice have been reported in prolonged high dose administration of synthetic testosterone, which gives credence to the use of the low dose regimens. Of course, natural testosterone is the recommended type of replacement. Two common preparations of natural testosterone are in a gel that is applied to the skin (transdermally) or in a tablet for use sublingually (under the tongue). When natural testosterone is swallowed, it is almost totally inactivated by the liver, therefore it is suggested that the transdermal or sublingual applications be used. Doses of testosterone do not have to be large in order to achieve the desired effects. Using lower doses helps prevent many of the unwanted side affects, which are extremely uncommon with natural testosterone. As with estrogen, transdermal application of testosterone gel is applied to areas of the body where the skin is generally thin and there is a rich supply of blood vessels, such as the abdomen, inner thighs, back of the hands and labia. It is recommended the sites of application be rotated daily. The gel must be allowed to remain on the skin at least 30 minutes for optimum absorption. The initial application should be in the morning, since the body's intrinsic testosterone level generally peaks in the morning, providing that much needed "get up and go." Should a second dose be required, it needs to be applied well before bedtime since some women experience insomnia from the inherent energizing effects of testosterone. Sublingual doses are timed the same as that for the gel form. It is best to start at conservative levels of replacement and monitor routinely to ensure that physiologic blood levels are achieved. Absorption by these methods of application is very rapid, with markedly elevated blood levels being achieved within hours, followed by a gradual decrease over the ensuing 6 to 8 hours. In order to get the natural hormone, a compounding pharmacist is needed. Dosages of 0.5 to 0.75 mg seem to be well tolerated while serving to relieve symptoms. Natural testosterone silastic capsules can be implanted beneath the skin, which is generally done in conjunction with estrogen replacement. Studies verify that blood levels of implanted testosterone are safe and remain stable for up to 6 months at a time. Finally, testosterone can be injected into the muscle in a "depo" form, but absorption following this route varies and thus limits its usefulness. This form of administration can also be painful.

SPEED NOTE

The most effective way to supplement testosterone is transdermally or sublingually, since natural testosterone, when swallowed in a pill form, is almost totally inactivated by the liver.

Currently, there are oral preparations of testosterone that have been chemically altered to permit passage through the liver without being destroyed. This is accomplished by "methylating" testosterone, which results in methyltestosterone. Estratest, which is a combined estrogen-methyltestosterone tablet, is approved for use in this country and contains 2.5 mg of methyltestosterone. It is unfortunate that blood tests for measuring methyltestosterone are not available. Breast tenderness, which is often noted with certain forms of estrogen therapy, can be decreased using methyltestosterone. Unlike natural testosterone, the methylated form does metabolize to estrogen, which can be an important consideration in breast cancer survivors. Whether natural or methylated testosterone is used, regular monitoring of liver function is recommended during hormone replacement therapy.

Thyroid Function

The thyroid gland, located in front of the throat below the Adam's apple, is important to female bodily functions. It regulates the rate at which the body utilizes oxygen while also controlling the functions of various organs and the speed with which the body utilizes food. As part of the "endocrine system," the thyroid acts as a thermostat by secreting hormones that enter the cells to regulate energy production. Imagine each of the cells in the body as a tiny microscopic power plant. It is up to the thyroid gland to signal the cell's engine to generate enough power or energy for normal cellular function. Without the thyroid, the body could not survive for very long!

A review of the physiology of the thyroid gland will provide an understanding to its importance. The two main thyroid hormones that regulate metabolic rate are thyroxin (T4) and triiodothyronine (T3). The thyroid secretes more T4 than T3 but most of the thyroid's activity is attributed to T3, which is five times more potent than T4. Formation of these hormones begins when iodine is absorbed by the intestines and is transported to the thyroid under the influence of a hormone called thyroid stimulating hormone (TSH). TSH is secreted by the pituitary gland in the brain and modulates the thyroid gland's production of T3 and T4, which then are released into the blood stream as thyroid hormones. T3 and T4 enter the cell to regulate the metabolic functions of energy production and building new tissue. Thus the thyroid gland is the principle gland that determines metabolic rate. The level of circulating T3 and T4 is critical for proper functioning of the body but it is also important that they have the ability to enter the cells and subsequently activate the cellular machinery. The majority of T3, the most potent, is made from T4 in tissues such as the liver and the kidneys. TSH secretion is controlled by the amount of circulating thyroid hormones in the blood stream.

SPEED NOTE

The thyroid gland determines the body's "metabolic rate" and signals the cell's engines to generate power or energy for cellular function. Without the thyroid, the body could not survive for very long.

Evaluation of thyroid function is based on symptoms and on blood tests. As with the ovaries, women in mid-life can begin a gradual decline in thyroid function that may not be reflected in blood tests alone. Blood tests assess circulating thyroid hormone levels of TSH and T4, but not necessarily the intracellular activity of T3 and T4, which are most important. Overt or severe thyroid problems can be diagnosed by these tests but it may take years before mild to moderate gland abnormalities produce abnormal blood tests.

Thyroid function is of particular importance for the woman in mid-life and beyond. Women have an increased incidence of hypothyroidism 10 times more frequently when compared to men. It has been estimated that 40% of women may manifest deficient thyroid function. Just as with the ovaries and adrenals, aging can cause a gradual decline in thyroid hormone production with resultant troubling symptoms. Hypothyroidism (insufficient production or absorption of thyroid hormone) rarely is seen in a severe form but instead is often manifested in its mild to moderate form. Symptoms of mild to moderate thyroid deficiency include 1) a general lack of energy 2) mental sluggishness 3) emotional instability 4) mood swings 5) intolerance to cold, especially of the hands and feet 6) dry, coarse, pale skin 7) coarse brittle hair 8) constipation 9) susceptibility to viral and respiratory infections and 10) irregular menstrual cycles. In past years, these changes have erroneously been attributed to aging. An important consideration is that the pre and post-menopausal decline in ovarian hormone production can also produce similar symptoms, but simply treating with hormones such as estrogen, progesterone and testosterone may not be enough. The thyroid gland should always be considered and evaluated.

SPEED NOTE

Thyroid hormone deficiencies can produce symptoms similar to ovarian hormone deficiencies. The thyroid should always be evaluated during hormone replacement therapy.

CHAPTER 6

THE IMPACT OF NUTRITION

Proper nutrition plays a vital role in maintaining optimal health. This is true not only for the menopausal woman, but for every human being. The demands for certain nutrients during menopause are extremely high and one consequence of deficiencies is hormonal imbalance.[7] The diet and lifestyle of our ancestors more readily met the nutritional needs of women than the typical diet and lifestyle of today. Several centuries ago few women had iron or vitamin B-12 deficiencies, and few suffered from degenerative diseases. Before World War II, processed food was the exception, not the rule. Food was fresh, full of nutrients and pesticide free. Awareness of the need for good nutrition in the management of menopause is increasing. A more in depth look at the role nutrition plays at the cellular level will demonstrate the importance of nutrition and how it relates to minimizing or preventing many of the problems related to the aging process and menopause.

---

[7] P.Choay, J.L. Lafond, A. Favier, *Value of Micronutrient Supplements in the Prevention or Correction of Disorders of Menopause,* Revue Francaise de Gynecologie et D Obstertrique, 1990: 85(12): 702.

Basic Cell Composition And Nutrition

Basic cell nutrition is critical. It is imperative that each individual cell be provided balanced nutrients in a bio-available form so that proper cell regeneration, function and communication can take place. As noted earlier, proper cell function and communication are critical in successfully managing hormone fluctuations and menopause. Cells are the smallest structures capable of basic life processes, such as the taking in of nutrients, expelling waste and reproducing. Cells carry out thousands of bio-chemical reactions each minute and reproduce new cells that perpetuate life. Cells form tissues (a group of similarly structured cells), tissues form organs (heart, stomach, brain), organs form organ systems (circulatory, digestive, nervous) and organ systems form the body. Therefore, the health of any one part of the body is determined by the health of the component cells.

Cells are composed of molecules, such as proteins, carbohydrates, fats and nucleic acid. Nucleic acid includes the DNA and RNA of the cell. The DNA is the cell's information library or command center containing hereditary information and instructions for cell regeneration. The RNA works in conjunction with the cell's DNA to build the proteins needed by each cell. The demand for protein in a cell never ceases. Cytoplasm, which is the semi-fluid that fills the cell, is about 65% water and is packed with about a billion molecules per cell. The cytoplasm is a virtual storehouse for enzymes and dissolved nutrients. The powerhouse of the cell is the mitochondria. This is where enzymes convert glucose and other nutrients into ATP (adenosine triphoshate) which serves as the energy for a wide variety of cell functions, including transferring substances across the plasma membrane, building and moving of proteins and lipids, recycling molecules and dividing cells. Without this energy, cell function would cease. All cells require nutrients and enzymes to be able to produce this energy. These nutrients and enzymes, most obtained from digested food, are supplied to the cells from the small intestines.

SPEED NOTE

Cells require nutrients and enzymes, mostly obtained from food, to provide the energy needed to carry out the thousands of functions completed each minute.

Enzymes

Enzymes are arguably the most important nutritional discovery since vitamins, minerals and trace elements, and perhaps one of the only solutions to our present health crisis. Enzymes are found in every living organism and without them life cannot continue. Enzymes are the work force, often times called the life force, of the human body. Enzymes are required for every chemical action and reaction in the body, including cell reproduction, metabolism, growth, digestion, hormone balancing, etc.[8] Without enzymes the mitochondira could not produce ATP, the energy for cell function. Without enzymes, neither vitamins, minerals, hormones nor any other element in the body

[8] Humbart Santillo, MH, N.D., *Food Enzymes: The Missing Link To Radiant Health,* (Prescott: Hohm Press, 1993),1.

could perform their work.[9] The body has the ability to produce a finite number of enzymes, but it must be realized that these enzyme reserves are being depleted at an extremely rapid rate due to diet and environment. Therefore, to maintain health as well as life, dense food enzymes must be ingested to support and replenish the body's enzyme reserves. In 1993 there were just over 1300 enzymes identified. As of today, the number is approaching 4,000.[10] It is significant to note that enzyme research is truly in its infancy, and it is expected that there will be substantially more identifiable enzymes isolated in the future.

The American Cancer Society and the American Heart Association recommend 5 to 9 servings of fresh raw fruits and vegetables be consumed daily to prevent disease. Yet, most people don't even come close to meeting these guidelines. And those who consume what they consider to be their daily requirement are frequently missing the most important part of the recommendation — fresh raw! Produce cooked, canned or processed in any other way is not the same as fresh raw. The reason — enzymes!

Initially, there must be a basic understanding that enzymes can only be formed from living matter, and when produce is harvested from the vine, the living matter is eliminated.[11] Therefore, no further enzyme development can take place. The mature enzyme, with the highest maximum density, is the best choice

---

[9] Dr. Edward Howell, *Food Enyzmes For Health and Longevity,* (Twin Lakes: Lotus Press, 1994), 17.
[10] D.A. Lopez, MD, M. Miehlke, MD, *Enzymes-The Fountain Of Life,* (Charleston: The Neville Press, Inc., 1994),1.
[11] Ibid., 1.

for the greatest impact and use in the body. The best source of mature enzymes is from vine-ripened fruits and vegetables. Keep in mind when shopping that most produce is not picked at the peak of ripeness; allowances are made for transit time, unpacking and shelf life. Much of the produce available at the grocery store was picked green, before full enzyme development could take place, resulting in underdeveloped enzymes and a lessened effect and impact in the body.

SPEED NOTE

Enzymes are the life force of the body and without enzymes life could not continue. The best source of dense enzyme nutrition comes from vine-ripened raw fruits and vegetables.

There are two groups of enzymes, exogenous (those consumed) and endogenous (those secreted or produced within the body). It is significant to note that enzyme balance and nutrient balance are required for optimal health. Enzymes are categorized into three classes: food, digestive and metabolic.[12] Food enzymes are exogenous, acquired from the food we eat. Found only in fresh raw food, they assist the digestive process. Categories of food enzymes include 1) lipase, which breaks down fat 2) protease, which breaks down

[12] Dr. Edward Howell, *Enzyme Nutrition,* (Wayne: Avery Publishing Group, 1985), 3.

proteins 3) amylase, which breaks down starches and 4) cellulase, which breaks down cellulose.[13] Technically, digestion begins in the mouth when food is chewed and the digestive enzymes found in saliva begin to break down carbohydrates.[14]

Metabolic enzymes work in the blood, the tissues and the organs. They are not obtained from raw food and cannot be effectively added to the system through supplementation. These endogenous enzymes are part of the enzyme reserve inherited at birth.[15] These are critical enzymes for life, supporting the brain, heart, kidney, liver, lungs, muscles, organs, glands and tissues. However, these metabolic enzymes also know that the body needs to have digested food to stay alive and will sacrifice themselves for digestive work if needed, instead of performing the catalytic reactions required in other parts of the body. Deficiencies in food and/or digestive enzymes will deplete the body's metabolic enzyme reserve. This means the life force is being taken away from these vital organs and tissues to facilitate the process of digestion. How can a strained muscle be repaired without an enzyme to channel the necessary reaction? How is the liver to properly cleanse the blood without appropriate enzymes? How can the lungs supply oxygen to the blood if there is not a sufficient level of enzymes to catalyze the reaction? In the menopausal woman, how

---

[13] Anthony J. Chichoke, DC, *Enzymes & Enzyme Therapy: How To Jump Start Your Way To Lifelong Good Health,* (New Canaan: Keats Publishing, 1994), 15.

[14] Dr. Edward Howell, *Food Enzymes For Health and Longevity,* (Twin Lakes: Lotus Press, 1994), 167.

[15] Humbart Santillo, MH, ND, *Food Enzymes: The Missing Link To Radiant Health,* (Prescott: Hohm Press, 1993),7.

can the endocrine system maintain hormone balances without the proper enzymes to perform the necessary reactions? To avoid jeopardizing the vital metabolic enzyme reserve, more fresh raw fruits and vegetables must be consumed on a daily basis.

Even though it is a powerful molecule, the enzyme is fragile when it comes to maintaining the ability to be a catalyst. Cooking, freezing, canning, microwaving or irradiating will denature the enzyme and it will no longer be capable of providing any catalytic benefit to the body. Enzymes do wear out and are dismantled by other enzymes and eliminated. Enzymes are lost through sweat, urine, feces and digestive fluids, consequently a constant supply of new food enzymes should be consumed daily.[16] Unfortunately, food choices today have more to do with convenience and taste than with nutritional value. Pre-menopause symptoms are often worsened if the body is chemically out of balance due to poor nutrition and improper lifestyle habits.[17] Studies indicate that symptoms of PMS may completely disappear when a nutrient dense diet is maintained.[18] Proper nutrition is vital in keeping a balanced endocrine system. So what happens when food is consumed?

[16] Humbart Santillo, MH, ND, *Intuitive Eating,* (Prescott: Hohm Press, 1993), 98.
[17] Anne Gittleman, *Super Nutrition For Menopause,* (New York: Pocket Books, 1993), 18.
[18] Betty Kamen, Ph.D., *Hormone Replacement Therapy – Yes or No?,* (Novato: Nutrition Encounter, 1996), 9.

SPEED NOTE

Metabolic enzymes that work in the blood, the tissues and the organs will be used for digestion if food and/or digestive enzymes are depleted. To protect the metabolic enzyme reserve, enzyme dense vine ripened fruits and vegetables must be consumed daily.

Antioxidants

Fresh raw fruits and vegetables also provide an excellent source of antioxidants. One role of antioxidants in the body is to neutralize waste by-products, known as free radicals, before irreparable damage has been done. Converting nutrients into energy for the body's use and other normal cellular functions will produce free radicals. These molecules have given up an electron during cell function, rendering them incomplete. A chain reaction begins to occur as the free radicals try to steal an electron from, or donate an electron to, other molecules, creating new free radicals. Key cellular components of the body, including DNA (the genetic blueprint in every cell), can be damaged during this process. Antioxidants stop this damaging chain reaction that can lead to cataracts, heart disease, cancer, arthritis and other degenerative diseases. Emotional stress can also be a cause of excess free radical production due to the higher levels of adrenaline being metabolized. Neutralizing and eliminating excess free radicals can result in symptoms that could include fatigue, intestinal problems, excess mucus secretion (runny nose and/or eyes) and body aches. Maintaining high levels of antioxidants is a significant component in maintaining healthy cells. Vitamin C, beta-carotene and vitamin E are all well researched antioxidants. More recently the identification of the antioxidants leutein, xeaxanthin (both found to target free radicals in the macula of the eye) and lycopene (reported to help prevent prostate cancer) would indicate that there are abundant nutrients in whole food that have not yet been discovered.

SPEED NOTE

Antioxidants found in fresh raw fruits and vegetables neutralize cell damaging free radicals and help to protect the system from developing degenerative diseases.

When unhealthy foods are consumed, the adrenals are placed under stress and begin to hyper-function. Looking at a typical diet, it is safe to say that the vast majority of women do not eat a truly healthy balanced diet. Years of improper nutrition, stress and environmental toxins take a toll on the system. By the time menopause is reached, without proper nutrition, the adrenals are either in a state of constant hyper-function or in burn-out! Amazingly, many of the same symptoms of hyper-functioning adrenals are also attributed to menopause (e.g. high blood pressure, headaches, hot flashes, excessive facial hair, etc.)[19] The adrenal glands supply estrone to the sys-

[19] Ann Gittleman, *Super Nutrition For Menopause,* (New York: Pocket Books, 1993), 18.

tem as the ovaries begin to slow their manufacture of estradiol and studies indicate that the healthier the adrenal glands, the fewer the menopause symptoms.[20] The evidence leads back to the importance of proper nutrition for a comfortable menopause.

There are, of course, some basic guidelines, but each woman must adapt the most healthy and nutritious diet for her lifestyle. It is obvious more food enzymes and antioxidants need to be consumed to maintain proper cell nutrition as well as for the preservation of the metabolic enzymes responsible for the hormonal activities in the endocrine system. Both antioxidants and enzymes are found in abundance in fresh raw fruits and vegetables.

Women seldom consume adequate amounts or sufficient varieties of fresh produce. Frequently what is consumed has been treated with pesticides and other chemicals containing substances known as xenoestrogens or xenobiotics that are endocrine destructive. The endocrine system is already under extreme stress during the menopause process; therefore, it is critical that these substances be avoided. These destructive chemicals are also found in solvents, plastics, glues, processed and synthesized foods, bug sprays, feed-lot meats and milk. To avoid these substances, organic products should be consumed whenever possible.

[21] John Robbins, *Diet For A New America*, (Walpole: Stillpoint Publishing, 1998), 191.

SPEED NOTE

Food consumed, especially fresh produce, should be organically grown so that endocrine destructive chemicals can be avoided. Solvents, plastics, glues, processed foods and bug sprays may contain these destructive substances.

It is apparent that a diet consisting of a wide variety of fresh raw fruits and vegetables, organically grown would be the ideal choice for the pre-menopausal woman. There are, however, other nutritional conditions to evaluate.

Calcium & Protein

Calcium and protein are critical nutrients for all women, no matter what stage of life. There is widespread confusion about the actual needs as well as how best to meet them. Recommendations abound involving dairy products as the best source of calcium supplementation. However, research shows that countries consuming the most dairy products have the highest incidence of osteoporosis. This is due in part to the excess dairy protein, which inhibits the absorption of calcium.[21] In addition, the body absorbs calcium inefficiently requiring additional amounts be consumed.[22] Companion nutrients including phospho-

[21] John Robbins, *Diet For A New America*, (Walpole: Stillpoint Publishing, 1998), 191.
[22] Sydney Lou Bonnick, MD, F.A.C.P., *The Osteoporosis Handbook*, (Dallas: Taylor Publishing Co., 1994),27.

rus, magnesium, vitamin D, silicon and boron are also required to facilitate proper calcium absorption. Individual daily requirements for calcium vary making it impossible to get the exact daily dose by ingesting multiple calcium and companion nutrient supplements. However, nature has an excellent and perfectly balanced solution. Dark green leafy vegetables such as spinach, kale, and romaine lettuce are packed with calcium as well as the companion nutrients required to maximize calcium absorption. The body will absorb more calcium from a salad made with spinach, romaine lettuce and summer vegetables than from standard doses of most calcium supplements on the market.

There are other diet-related factors that obstruct the absorption of calcium. Sugar, salt, protein, processed meats, caffeine and tobacco all inhibit calcium absorption. These inhibitors leave "acidic ash" in the system and calcium works as one of the neutralizing minerals that transform the acidic ash into an alkaline ash so that it can be eliminated.[23] Fruits and vegetables leave an alkaline ash in the system that can be eliminated efficiently and will also leave mineral deposits in the system to help neutralize acidic ash.[24] Further confusing the calcium story is research indicating that a low protein diet combined with limiting the above mentioned calcium inhibitors is the most effective way to restore a positive calcium balance.[25]

---

[23] Gary Null, *The Complete Guide To Health & Nutrition,* (New York: Dell Publishing, 1984), 30.
[24] Ibid.
[25] John A. McDougall, MD and Mary McDougall, *The McDougall Plan,* (Clinton: New Win Publishing, Inc., 1993), 100-101.

SPEED NOTE

Calcium is better absorbed from foods such as spinach, kale and romaine lettuce than from supplements. Limiting sugar, salt, protein, processed meats, caffeine, alcohol and tobacco will allow calcium to be better absorbed in the body.

Protein is an essential part of a healthy diet and proper cell function, but there are many opinions as to the necessary amount of protein that should be consumed. The general recommendations suggest 40 grams per day of protein intake for the average woman. A diet that contains more than one serving of meat (the most concentrated protein) per day could easily exceed this recommended intake amount.[26] A high protein diet can actually cause calcium to be leached from bones to neutralize the abundant acidic ash.

There are many know and unknown ingredients working synergistically to maintain the body's chemical balance. Supplementing only the known ingredients can upset this delicate balance. Food should be the main source of nutrition for the body because nature has uniquely balanced the nutritional content of whole food. Processing food, either by steaming, boiling, freezing, canning or microwaving can result in a substantial loss of critical nutritional elements. Research indicates that consuming a wide variety of

[26] Sydney Lou Bonnick, MD, F.A.C.P., *The Osteoporosis Handbook,* (Dallas: Taylor Publishing Company, 1994), 16.

nutritiously dense whole food will provide a more complete spectrum of vital nutrients.

Sugars & Carbohydrates

Keeping the body in chemical balance includes maintaining relatively constant blood sugar levels. Depression, mood swings, anxiety, headaches and fatigue that are frequently experienced through the menopause process are often intensified by fluctuations in blood sugar levels. A proper diet and avoiding high glycemic and high simple carbohydrate foods can help maintain a proper balance.

The ability of a food to raise glucose in the blood is known as its "glycemic index." The glycemic index of food is measured against glucose (with an index number of 100) because glucose has the greatest and fastest ability to raise blood sugar levels. The higher the index number the faster the rise and subsequent fall in blood sugar. The glycemic index chart at the end of this chapter will provide examples of foods and their corresponding index numbers based on their comparative ability and speed in boosting blood sugars. It is interesting to not that fructose, the simple sugar found in fruits and vegetables, has a lower index number (at 20) than a potato (at 70) or corn flakes (at 80). Carrots have an extremely high index number of 92.

Glucose is used for energy in the cell and insulin is the regulator. In muscle insulin facilitates glucose uptake, stimulates its conversion to glycogen and increases protein. In fatty tissue insulin facilitates the conversion of glucose to fatty acids. Insulin levels are affected by glucose; excess insulin disrupts hormonal communications including those associated with menopause and the control of fat storage.

> ***<u>SPEED NOTE</u>***
>
> ***Foods that raise blood sugar levels will adversely affect hormone communication. Avoid simple carbohydrates and high glycemic foods.***

Bone Density & Osteoporosis

It is widely publicized that estrogen protects bones, and from that a misconception has developed that estrogen actually builds bones. That is not the case. Estrogen protects against bone loss by reducing the activity of osteoclasts, cells that take calcium from the bone.[27] A supply of calcium must always be present in the blood for nerve cell communication, contraction of muscle, blood-clotting efficiency, enzyme function and production of life supporting proteins.[28] The osteoclast will take calcium from the bone to keep the levels in the blood in an optimal range. Estrogen reduces the activity of the osteoclasts and consequently there is a reduction in the leaching of calcium from the bones.

Progesterone works in conjunction with osteoblasts, cells that are associated with building new bone.[29] Progesterone could actively increase bone

---

[27] Betty Kamen, Ph.D., *Hormone Replacement Therapy-Yes or No?*, (Navato: Nutrition Encounter, 1993), 110.
[28] Ibid., 81.
[29] Ibid., 110.

mass and density which could prevent or even reverse osteoporosis.[30] Bone is living matter and it is never too late to begin rebuilding it. Due to a diet lacking in many nutrients, signs of osteoporosis are being seen as early as age 20. There is a need to heed this as a definite warning signal to focus on nutritional needs with a much greater intensity prior to menopause.

Weight bearing exercise is an important key often overlooked in the process of rebuilding and protecting bone density. The perception that "weight bearing exercise" can only be accomplished through lengthy sessions at the gym "pumping iron" has kept many women inactive. A 20-30 minute daily brisk walk provides one of the most beneficial overall exercises for the prevention of osteoporosis. The endorphins released by a brisk walk can help relieve many symptoms, including depression and sleep problems, in the pre-menopausal woman. It is important to note that with advanced osteoporosis care must be given to avoid excessive force or weight that could increase the risk of bone fracture.

SPEED NOTE

The best exercise to help rebuild and protect bone density is brisk walking. Bones are living matter and can be rebuilt.

[30] John R. Lee, MD, *What Your Doctor May Not Tell You About Menopause,* (New York: Warner Books, 1996) 160.

Water

It is important to drink fresh, pure, chemical free water every day to promote and maintain cellular health. With over 70% of the body being made up of water it is easy to comprehend why water is so vital to life. Well hydrated cells are healthier cells because water not only carries nutrients to each cell, it also removes the wastes and toxins from each cell. Without sufficient water cells become clogged and sluggish with waste material and elimination problems can become troublesome.

Regular municipal tap water, like many of the processed foods, can actually be detrimental to health because of the presence of chlorine. Chlorine can mimic estrogen in the body and has been linked to various forms of breast cancer.[31] Like other xenoestrogens discussed earlier, chlorine can be ingested or absorbed into the body. During a 20-minute shower with public supplied tap water, the body can absorb the same amount of chlorine that would be ingested in a gallon of that tap water.[32] A water filtration system is ideal to eliminate chlorine before using or drinking it. If chlorinated tap water is the only choice, take the extra time to disburse the chlorine before drinking the water. Fill a pitcher with water and let it stand uncovered for 24 hours, and most of the chlorine will have dissipated.[33]

---

[31] Derrick M. DeSilva Jr., MD, *Ask The Doctor,* (Loveland: Interweave Press, 1997), 126.
[32] Ibid.
[33] Betty Kamen, Ph.D., *Hormone Replacement Therapy-Yes or No?,* (Novato: Nutrition Encounter, 1996), 144.

Fats

The importance of fruits and vegetables, the ingestion of calcium rich foods, the limitations of protein, the benefits of exercise and the necessity of water have all been reviewed. The next important dietary topic is fat. Every cell in the body requires fat as part of a balancing system for cell protection. A totally fat free diet is not the answer. There are fats that should be avoided and there are fats that are beneficial and should be included as part of a healthy diet.

Monounsaturated fats, found in olive oil, olives, avocados, almonds, peanuts, pecans, cashews and pistachio nuts, can actually provide benefits to the system by lowering LDL (bad) cholesterol without lowering HDL (good) cholesterol. Omega-3 fatty acids are found in salmon, herring, anchovies, dark green leafy vegetables and soy beans. Omega-3 fatty acids can help lower LDL cholesterol and actually increase HDL cholesterol. Fish is an ideal menu choice several times a week, provided it is broiled, grilled or sautéed — just don't fry it!

Polyunsaturated fats are found in vegetable oils, sunflower seeds and some nuts, including walnuts, Brazil nuts and pine nuts. In excess, this type of fat may lower HDL (good) cholesterol, and may promote artery-blocking plaque buildup and increase cancer risks. Limited intake of polyunsaturated fat is favorable. Saturated fat, found in high fat meats, ground beef, high fat dairy products and tropical oils like coconut oil, can also lead to plaque in the arteries. Saturated fat also increases LDL (bad) cholesterol, which raises the risk of heart disease. Avoidance or extremely limited ingestion of saturated fat is recommended.

The fat that should be totally avoided is trans-fat, or hydrogenated fat. This type of fat, found in margarine, especially stick form, and crisp processed foods like cookies, crackers and chips, increases LDL levels, decreases HDL levels, thus increasing the risk of heart attack and stroke. Hydrogenated fats act like Styrofoam in the blood, clogging the system. It is imperative to learn to read the ingredients labels on foods purchased and avoid hydrogenated fats completely.

SPEED NOTE

Some fat is beneficial to the system. Monounsaturated fat, found in olives, avocados, and some nuts, and Omega-3 fatty acids, found in cold water fish, dark green leafy vegetables and soybeans, should comprise the majority of fat ingested. Polyunsaturated fat, found in vegetable oils and some nuts, should be limited. The fats to avoid are saturated fat and hydrogenated fat.

The information contained in this chapter will supply basic guidelines to follow for a smoother transition into menopause. The primary focus for obtaining optimal health is to maintain healthy cells. Adopt healthy nutritional habits immediately. Stop "dieting" and focus on lifestyle changes that will result in long term permanent benefits. When such strong emphasis is placed on weight loss, women get caught in an endless cycle of fad diets that may allow quick weight loss but not proper nutrition. Instead of weight loss as a primary goal, the focus must be on taking charge of nutritional choices available — fresh whole foods, chemical free water, exercise and balance.

The following food charts are designed to provide assistance in food choices. A balanced diet is the healthiest diet. Stay in control of the hand to mouth motion. The better a woman's overall health, the easier the transition will be through menopause. That alone is worth the effort.

FOOD CHART EXPLANATIONS

The first charts indicate the amounts of calcium, phosphorus and silicon in some common foods. These minerals are part of the necessary elements needed for bone building. The recommended daily intake of calcium is 1000 mg. and phosphorus intake should be only slightly higher than that. Increased calcium consumption demands an increase in magnesium rich foods for proper absorption. There is a separate chart for foods high in magnesium. There are no current dietary guidelines for silicon or boron intake, and there is limited information about food contents of these minerals. Soil conditions and absorption rates of these minerals vary greatly so two bunches of spinach could have dramatically different contents of silicon and boron. However, these are vital nutrients required for building bones, therefore it is advised to eat a wide variety of fruits and vegetables.

CALCIUM, PHOSPHORUS & SILICON VALUES
MEASURED IN MG. PER 100 GRAM SERVING (APPROX. 4 OZ.)

VEGETABLES

Food	Calcium	Phosphorus	Silicon
Alfalfa	1754	251	0
Asparagus	21	50	2
Beans, Kidney	46	91	2
Beans, String	50	37	2
Beets	14	23	88
Broccoli	88	62	22
Brussel Sprouts	32	72	2
Cabbage	130	230	9
Carrots	37	36	22
Cauliflower	25	56	33
Celery	39	28	31
Chard	81	36	7
Cucumbers	26	28	35
Kale	249	73	2
Lettuce, Romaine	68	25	40
Parsley	204	63	38
Peas, Fresh	23	99	2
Potatoes, Sweet	40	58	20
Spinach	93	38	181

CALCIUM, PHOSPHORUS & SILICON VALUES
MEASURED IN MG. PER 100 GRAM SERVING (APPROX. 4 OZ.)

FRUITS

Food	Calcium	Phosphorus	Silicon
Apples	7	10	64
Apricots	17	34	53
Avocado	10	42	11
Bananas	8	26	20
Blueberries	15	13	0
Cantaloupe	14	16	88
Cherries	22	19	66
Cranberries	124	20	2
Dates	59	63	2
Figs	124	76	35
Lemons	17	11	35
Olives	106	17	7
Oranges	41	20	4
Papaya	35	104	4
Peaches	9	19	2
Pears	8	11	7
Strawberries	21	21	22
Tangerines	30	13	1
Watermelon	7	10	11

CALCIUM & PHOSPHORUS VALUES

MEASURED IN MG PER 100 GRAM SERVING (APPROX. 4 OZ.)

MEATS	Calcium	Phosphorus
Bacon	14	224
Beef, Roast	11	140
Bologna	7	128
Chicken, Roast	11	265
Chicken, Fried	13	272
Corned Beef	9	93
Frankfurter	5	102
Ham	9	172
Hamburger	22	141
Pork Chops	10	232
Steak, T-Bone	10	186
Turkey	11	300
FISH & SEAFOOD		
Crabmeat	43	174
Flounder, baked	23	349
Halibut, broiled	16	252
Kelp	1093	240
Salmon	258	342
Sardines, canned	272	432
Shrimp	72	190
Tuna, canned	8	233

CALCIUM & PHOSPHORUS VALUES
MEASURED IN MG. PER 100 GRAM SERVING (APPROX. 4 OZ.)

GRAINS

	Calcium	Phosphorus
Bran Flakes	53	358
Brown Rice	12	73
Cornflakes	16	32
Farina, instant	77	60
Graham Crackers	40	143
Oatmeal	9	58
Shredded Wheat	43	389
Wheat Germ	48	1085
Wheat Bran	119	1121
White Bread	100	115
White Rice	10	28
Whole Wheat Flour	41	372

EGGS & DAIRY

	Calcium	Phosphorus
Cheese, Cheddar	753	476
Cheese, Cream	94	152
Egg, Boiled	54	206
Milk, Skim	121	95
Milk, Whole	118	93
Yogurt, Low-Fat	120	94

CALCIUM & PHOSPHORUS VALUES

MEASURED IN MG. PER 100 GRAM SERVING (APPROX. 4 OZ.)

MISCELLANEOUS

	Calcium	Phosphorus
Almonds	234	504
Blackstrap Molasses	685	85
Cashews	39	373
French Salad Dressing	11	14
Grapefruit Juice	8	14
Italian Dressing	10	4
Light Molasses	165	45
Maple Syrup	105	8
Minestrone Soup	15	24
Peanut Butter	57	380
Peanuts, Roasted	75	401
Sunflower Seeds	120	837
Tomato Juice	7	18
Walnut	0	570

MAGNESIUM VALUES

MEASURED IN MG. PER 100 GRAM SERVING (APPROX. 4 OZ.)

Food	Magnesium
Almonds	270
Avocados	31
Bananas	30
Barley	55
Brazil Nuts	220
Cashews	27
Chard	65
Cheese, Cheddar	29
Coconut	40
Corn	37
Molasses, Blackstrap	410
Molasses, Light	81
Oats	140
Pecans	140
Pistachios	160
Rice, Brown	120
Salmon	38
Soybeans	240
Spinach	57
Sunflower Seeds	350
Tuna, canned	27
Turkey	44
Walnuts	130
Wheat Germ	320

Selecting foods with lower glycemic index numbers will support a more stable blood sugar reading. Remember this is ONLY a guide. This is not stating that all foods with higher ratings should be avoided, just limited. The chart below is to provide basic information and guidelines.

GLYCEMIC INDEX CHART

Ratings based on approximate serving size of 4 oz.

Food	Index	Food	Index
Apple	39	Orange, fresh	40
All-Bran	51	Orange Juice	46
Bananas	62	Parsnips	97
Beets	64	Peanuts	13
Black-eyed Peas	33	Potato Chips	51
Brown Rice	66	Raisins	64
Carrots	90	Soybeans	15
Cornflakes	80	Spaghetti, Wheat	42
Honey	87	Spaghetti, White	60
Kidney Beans	29	Sweet Corn	59
Lentils	29	Sweet Potatoes	48
Lima Beans	36	Wheat Bread	72
Milk, Skim	32	White Bread	69
Milk, Whole	34	White Potatoes	70

CHAPTER 7

HORMONE SUPPLEMENTS (A Review)

With the discovery that female hormone management is a complex series of interactions between various glands, organs and bio-chemical reactions, we should evaluate the choices available when it comes to symptom treatment and managing individual health from pre-menopause, through menopause and finally into post-menopause. Focusing primarily on the types of progesterone and estrogen supplementation available, be sure to discuss options and concerns with a professional health care provider to ensure receipt of the greatest benefit from the chosen therapy.

Natural progesterone is a female sex hormone that is also found in males. Due to the elevated instance of adverse side affects of synthetic progestins, starting with a natural form is highly recommended. Natural progesterone has not only been recommended for pre- and post- menopausal women, but also for problems such as amenorrhea (absence of menstruation), dysmenorrhea (painful menstruation), endometriosis and premenstrual tension.

The most common form of natural progesterone is that found in topical creams, many of which contain some form of Mexican Wild Yam. Applying the cream on the skin allows the progesterone to bypass the liver. This is one of the most beneficial reasons to use a transdermal application. What is the difference between natural progesterone and Mexican Wild Yam? This is a very important point to consider when evaluating the brand of "natural progesterone" to be used. The selected health care provider may have some specific band name recommendations. However, if that is not the case, look specifically for a cream that is labeled to contain "natural progesterone." This is the lab converted derivative of the Mexican Wild Yam. The label may also read "Activated Wild Yam," which means it has been converted to natural progesterone. Many creams contain just the Mexican Wild Yam, which the body cannot convert into progesterone. Also, be aware of creams containing "U.S.P. grade progesterone," since this is not from a natural source and is not as biocompatible with the body. Likewise avoid creams that contain only diosgenin, also called "wild yam extract." This is a chemical derived from the Mexican Wild Yam, but the molecular structure is too large to be effectively absorbed through the skin.

There are other factors to consider as well when selecting a topical progesterone. When making the first brand selection it is imperative to read the ingredients label very carefully. Taking this extra time will result in obtaining a higher quality product to use. Previously discussed was the avoidance of xenoestrogens or xenobiotics due to their endocrine destructive ability. Some brands of natural progesterone use these petrochemical substances, often labeled as "propylene glycol," as the base for the cream. Avoid these creams completely! There are other preservatives that should be avoided as well, if at all possible; some ingredients are known as parabens (propyl, methyl, butly, or ethyl), benzene, cetyl alcohol and polysorbate 60.

SPEED NOTE

Natural progesterone is most commonly found in a topical cream. Care should be taken in selecting a brand of natural progesterone so that optimal absorption can take place and to avoid harmful preservatives and additives.

Now that the variety of creams available have been evaluated, selection of a brand meeting the above criteria begins. *Progesta-Care* and *Premier Natural Gesterone Cream* are two good choices and are found at most quality health food stores. There is some concern, although not thoroughly documented, that the progesterone effectiveness of creams packaged in the jars may deteriorate from daily exposure to oxygen, or that the cream may become contaminated with daily exposure to the hands. Creams in tubes or pump bottles are often recommended. If the jar container is all that is available in the brand selected to meet the criteria, get the jar!

Now that the progesterone cream selection has been made, how is it used? Primary application sites are the wrists, inside upper arms, breasts and neck, where the skin is quite thin. Secondary sites are the stomach, buttocks and inner thigh. It is advisable and highly recommended to rotate the application sites to avoid saturation of one area.[34] Application of cream should be done twice a day, remembering to alternate the application sites. How much of a specific brand cream to be used will depend on the individual needs as well as the assimilation of the natural progesterone. Most brands advise using 1/4 – 1/2 teaspoon twice daily. The health care provider may recommend an alternative dose; however attention to the individual results obtained will be a critical indicator of whether adjustments will be needed for the application amounts. Optimal results may require experimentation with several brands of topical natural progesterone. Make note of all physical and symptom changes during this trial time.

There are other forms of natural progesterone as well. Oils, sublingual drops and capsules are available. The oils are applied transdermally, the same as the creams, but are often quite sticky. Sublingual drops are normally found in combination with vitamin E oil. Held under the tongue, absorption is allowed through the mucous membranes of the mouth. The levels of progesterone in the blood will increase rapidly then will fall within three to four hours. For this reason drops should be administered three to four times a day.[35] Capsules must contain higher dosages of natural progesterone to achieve the same affects as transdermal or sublingual applications, due to the fact that by ingesting the capsule, the body will first send it through the liver, which will eliminate ap-

[34] John R. Lee, MD, *What Your Doctor May Not Tell You About Menopause,* (New York: Warner Books, Inc., 1996), 266.
[35] Ibid.

proximately 85% of the dosage.[36] This process is called "first pass loss." For this reason capsule supplementation of progesterone is not recommended.

If, by chance, consideration is being given to the use of synthetic progestins, make sure the adverse side affects are thoroughly discussed with the health care provider. Two of the brand names are Provera and Norlutin. It is imperative that all the possible side affects be reviewed before deciding on synthetic progestins. Long term use of synthetic progestins is not recommended. Again, there are many choices, but ultimately, the final choice is that of the individual.

SPEED NOTE

Progesterone supplementation can be accomplished with natural or synthetic treatment. Natural progesterone topical creams are the safest and most often recommended therapy.

Now, examine estrogen supplementation and the various options available. The benefits of estrogen supplementation have been discussed in detail in Chapter 3. The three types of estrogen found in the body are estrone, estradiol, and estriol, each performing a different function. The fourth type of estrogen is synthetic. The most common synthetic estrogen in Premarin, previously discussed. This type has an altered molecular structure when compared to the

[36] Ibid.

body's natural estrogens, yet still has enough similarity in structure to be able to attach to various estrogen receptor sites. There are numerous natural and synthetic estrogen supplements available. Be advised that a complete evaluation by a professional health care provider is mandatory before beginning estrogen supplementation.

A very safe and effective way to add estrogen to the body is through phytoestrogens — those found in food. There have been no adverse affects reported from increasing the consumption of foods high in phytoestrogens. Of course, soy and all soy products, including tofu, miso, aburage, atuage, koridofu, and sprouted beans provide an excellent source of phytoestrogens. Other sources include black cohosh, alfalfa, licorice and pomegranates. It is advisable to add one or more of these foods to the diet every day. Even for those who have had breast cancer and are to avoid supplemental estrogen, these phytoestrogens can actually work to protect the estrogen receptor sites in the body. Phytoestrogens can be thought of as the "good" estrogen.

SPEED NOTE

Phytoestrogens, found in food, are the safest way to supplement estrogen.

The focus has been primarily on progesterone and estrogen, but there are other hormones in the body that are often sought out and taken for supplementation. DHEA (Dehydroepiandrosterone) is a major raw material for the hormone testosterone and estradiol. In some instances supplementation with DHEA can prove effective, but this should ***only*** be done after testing has shown an actual need for DHEA. Close observation by a professional health care provider is mandatory with DHEA supplementation. DHEA can actually increase the estrogen load in the body.[37] Another problem with DHEA is the fact that while there are many studies reporting all the positive affects, the negative results are frequently left out. For example, a study done at the University of California at San Diego reported that men with low DHEA levels had twice the incidence of heart disease and death as men whose DHEA levels were very high. What was ***not*** reported was that women with high levels of DHEA turned out to be at ***greater*** risk of heart disease than those whose levels were lower.[38] Also, an experiment with 16 rats showed that 14 developed liver cancer after supplementation with DHEA![39] The discussion of "first pass loss" through the liver explained that 85% of the hormones that were ingested were absorbed and cleansed through the liver before ever reaching the system. The corresponding results of the rats developing liver cancer would make sense. If DHEA were a drug and not a supplement, human testing would have been stopped! Supplementation with DHEA should be very carefully monitored. The long term ramifications are not yet known.

---

[37] Betty Kamen, Ph.D., *Hormone Replacement Therapy-Yes or No?,* (Novato: Nutrition Encounter, 1996) 41.
[38] Isadore Rosenfeld, MD, *Dr. Rosenfeld's Guide to Alternative Medicine,* (New York: Random House, 1996) 305.
[39] Ibid.

SPEED NOTE

All hormone supplementation, including hormones like DHEA, should be done under the supervision of a qualified health care provider.

Another hormone that is now available is testosterone. Again, this is not a hormone to supplement unless testing as well as symptom monitoring had been done to show an actual deficiency. Extremely low does of compounded testosterone can have very powerful, and sometimes unwanted, affects on the system. Excessive facial hair, acne and irritability are frequent complaints when incorrect dosages are taken. Insulin resistance has also been reported as a side affect of testosterone supplementation. Caution is recommended when taking a compounded testosterone, and notation of any physical changes should be reported to the health care provider.

The key to selecting the right supplementation for specific individual needs is to learn to listen to the signals from the body. Pay attention to subtle changes in moods, memory, energy levels, clarity of thinking, libido, etc. Note the positive and the negative, and report these to the health care provider. Communication is a very critical element when dealing with hormones and the effort put forth to regain balance. Herbs are another frequently used means of treating symptoms associated with hormonal fluctuations. Some of the most frequently used herbs are Dong Quai, Unicorn Root, Sarsparilla, Black Cohosh, Blue

Cohosh and Licorice. Dong Quai is most often used for irregular or difficult menstruation. It has been reported to help balance female hormone chemistry, although it does not have estrogen like activity. It is a good selection for mild hormone imbalances. Unicorn Root is not well researched. It does contain a form of diosgenin and appears to have some hormonal activity by seeming to alleviate some menopausal symptoms. Sarsparilla is a gentle stimulant for the adrenals. Keep in mind, many women who are entering menopause are doing so with hyper-functioning adrenal glands, and additional stimulation is not necessary. Sarsparilla has the structural similarity to human steroid hormones. Black Cohosh, a favorite herb to provide relief from hot flashes, is highly estrogenic. Although no specific studies have been completed, unopposed with progesterone, the risk of endometrial build-up and endometrial cancer could exist. A safer option would be Blue Cohosh. Demonstrating very similar properties, but less estrogenic, Blue Cohosh is a safer option if progesterone is not used. Licorice, although used frequently in Chinese medicine, has varied hormonal effects for women. Conclusive research is not available on the hormonal affects of Licorice. It is recommended that individuals with high blood pressure avoid the use of Licorice.

There are increasing numbers of health care providers who are open to including complementary approaches with allopathic practices. Whether you see an allopathic physician or a naturopath is chosen, education and communication are critical. Integration of these two fields of practice will eventually lead to better health care and treatment for everyone.

CHAPTER 8

THE DOCTOR'S PRESCRIPTION
(A Summary)

The purpose of this book is to provide an integrative approach to managing the aging process of the female endocrine system in an effort to achieve a better quality of life during this transitional time. It is also imperative to note that the process of integrating the allopathic and the naturopathic fields of medicine can be accomplished with amazingly positive results. The benefits of integrating both fields can provide positive results not only for women experiencing uncomfortable symptoms of menopause, but also for other types of conditions and illnesses.

Understanding what can and cannot be provided by each type of practice will furnish basic groundwork. The next step is to become aware of where to find guidance and education with regard to the choices available. Many people are now seeking alternative treatments for all types of illnesses, unfortunately, the search frequently produces more confusion than answers.

The understanding of genetics has provided vast knowledge in the areas of treatment and prevention of many chronic diseases. Although menopause is not a disease, it is a condition associated with the "wearing out" of the ovaries. Lifestyle changes have been a key factor in how women age. It must never be forgotten that lifestyle encompasses nutrition, exercise, stress reduction and gynecologic wellness. What is know is that today's woman has an increase in overall body weight, and earlier onset of puberty, less physical activity and exhibits a much poorer food selection. There have been more changes in the diet in the last 50 years than in all recorded human history. These dietary changes reflect an evolutionary process that is not working, that is readily apparent in the poor state of health in the vast majority of people. Proper nutrition is critical to cellular integrity which must be at optimal levels during all stages of life, especially menopause.

NUTRITION

(Review food tables in Chapter 6)

Proper Nutrition Does Not Come From A Multi-Vitamin Pill!

5 - 9 Servings Of Fresh Raw Fruits And Vegetables Per Day

Fruits and vegetables contain vital nutrients (vitamins, minerals, trace elements, and fiber) in a balanced synergistic form. When consumed raw, they are also a prime source of vital enzymes, required for maintaining life. It is recommended that the fruits and vegetables eaten raw should be organic to avoid any chemical ingestion. And, the wider the variety, the better the nutritional impact. Choose the deepest, darkest varieties to provide the most dense nutrition. Supplementing the diet with a whole food concentrate, such as Juice Plus+, is recommended.

Calcium

Calcium is required for bone building; however, just taking a supplement is not necessarily the best solution for increasing the body's calcium level. Research also indicates that dairy products may not be the best way to acquire more usable calcium, seemingly due to the excess amount of dairy protein. The proper absorption of calcium is based on many factors, including a balance of nutrients such as phosphorus, magnesium, silicon, boron and vitamin D. It is virtually impossible to attain this balance through vitamin supplements. The best alternative is to eat an abundance of green leafy vegetables, such as spinach, romaine lettuce, kale, turnip greens and swiss chard, which contain the co-factor nutrients necessary for optimal calcium absorption. Broccoli and parsley are also an excellent source of calcium. Calcium absorption inhibitors, such as sugar, salt, processed meats, excess protein, caffeine, alcohol and tobacco should be limited.

Protein

Protein is essential for proper cell function, but excess protein can produce other problems. The average woman should consume approximately 30-40 grams of protein per day, which could be found in one average serving of meat. The acidic ash that remains after protein is digested must be neutralized before elimination, and calcium is one of the minerals used to perform that function.

Glycemic Index

To keep the body chemistry in balance, the blood sugar levels must also stay relatively constant. Avoiding high glycemic and high simple carbohydrate foods will help maintain a more constant blood sugar level. The glycemic index chart in Chapter 6 lists the glycemic ratings on some common foods.

Water

Water is an important part of the nutritional picture, but is oftentimes forgotten. A minimum of 64 ounces of chemical free (purified or filtered) water per day is a requirement to maintain optimal health. Chlorine and other chemicals are toxins to the body and should be eliminated from the water consumed.

Fats

All fats are not bad. Proper cell function requires some fat, but it must be the right combination of fat. Beneficial fats are monounsaturated and Omega-3 fatty acids. Olive oil, olives, avocados, almonds, peanuts, pecans, cashews and pistachio nuts are all excellent sources of monounsaturated fats. Omega-3 fatty acids are found in fish (salmon, herring, sardines), dark green leafy vegetables and soy beans. These types of fats should be the source of daily fat intake. Polyunsaturated fats are found in vegetable oils, sunflower seeds and some nuts, and consumption of this type of fat should be limited. Saturated fat, found in high fat meats, high fat dairy and tropical oils should be greatly limited. The fats to avoid are trans-fats or hydrogenated fats, found in margarine and crisp processed foods.

EXERCISE

A study conducted at the University of Southern California reported that women who exercised 35 minutes a day reduced their risk of breast cancer by as much as 60%. According to a Harvard study, women who exercised vigorously just once a week had a 37% lower risk of diabetes than those who did not exercise. It has been stated that 50% of functional decline can be prevented through exercise. Proper exercise will support the cardiovascular system, help build bone density and lean muscle mass, increase HDL (good) cholesterol, decrease LDL (bad) cholesterol, lower blood pressure and release endorphins, a powerful mood lifting chemical produced by the body as a result of exercise. These benefits of exercise are important when dealing with menopause. Exercise exerts its beneficial effects on numerous organ systems, which will be discussed in a future publication.

HORMONES

Synthetic and Natural Choices

It is always advised to seek the direction of a professional health care provider before hormone supplementation begins. Testing should be conducted to more definitively determine which hormones need to be supplemented. There are two types of testing that can be performed. Blood tests have been the most common method of determining hormone levels, however, they can also be inaccurate. The blood may carry a biologically inactive portion of the hormones. A blood test may measure the inactive hormone as well as the active hormones resulting in an unreliable reading. Lab testing should always be accompanied by a thorough symptom analysis, which may expose neurohormonal deficiencies not commonly identified in lab results. Saliva testing is now available and is completed over a period of three to thirty days. Saliva testing may prove to be more accurate in determining active hormone levels, and thus provide better information on which to make hormone supplementation decisions.

Estrogen

Premarin has been the most widely prescribed non-human estrogen. Positive results in menopause symptom treatment have been achieved with Premarin. But, because it contains at least nine different conjugated estrogens not found in humans, the possible side affects could be quite dangerous. Synthetic non-human estrogens do not have the exact molecular structure of the hormone that the body produces. The structure is similar enough to be able to attach to the estrogen receptors throughout the body, but it is not an exact match. Whenever taking synthetic hormones make sure to evaluate all the potential side affects to determine if the benefits will outweigh the risks.

Anti-estrogens, Tamoxifen and Raloxifen, are non-human preparations that compete for estrogen receptor sites. These preparations are used in an effort to inhibit estrogen-sensitive tumor growth. Side affects should be reviewed carefully before taking an anti-estrogen.

Xenoestrogens are substances that have estrogenic effects, but are endocrine destructive. These substances are found in petrochemically derived products, such as pesticides, herbicides, plastics, solvents, glues, insect sprays, etc. Tobacco, alcohol and chlorine all produce these same endocrine destructive elements in the system. Exposure to these substances should be avoided.

Native or natural hormones have the exact molecular structure of the hormones the body produces. These type hormones should be the first choice in supplementation selection because they provide a safer method of estrogen replacement therapy. Estradiol, estrone and estriol are all native hormones and are now available. They can be administered in pill form to be swallowed, transdermally (applied to the skin), injected, implanted under the skin or taken sublingually (under the tongue). Synthetic hormones are derived from other than natural sources and do not have the exact molecular structure of the human hormone.

Phytoestrogens, or phytoesterols, are plant estrogens that are structurally and functionally similar to human estradiol. They are believed to attach to estrogen receptors preventing continued exposure to high levels of estrogen, and also may act as replacements for depleted hormones at menopause. These phytoestrogens can be found in flaxseed, whole grain cereals, vegetables, legumes, fruits, soy based products and chickpeas. There appears to be no adverse side effects associated with consumption of phytoestrogen rich food.

Progesterone

Synthetic progestins, such as Provera, are included in hormone replacement therapy to prevent uterine cancer as a result of estrogen replacement. The adverse side effects associated with synthetic progestins should be closely examined before a decision to use them is made.

Natural progesterone provides a safe and effective means to replenish a diminishing hormone. Transdermal application is the most popular method of supplementation. Select only creams that contain "natural progesterone" or "Activated Wild Yam". Avoid products with ingredient labels indicating "propylene glycol," "cetyl alcohol," or "parabens" in the cream. Experimentation with several brands of progesterone cream may be necessary. Natural progesterone is also available in oils, sublingual drops and capsules.

HERBS

There are many herbs and herb combination products on the market that claim to provide relief from menopausal symptoms. Some will work and some will not. The most popular, and the most recommended herbs used for symptom relief are Blach Cohosh, Blue Cohosh and Dong Quai. The symptom relieving effects of herbs may take up to four weeks to be noticed. Patience is important when using herbs for supplementation.

The dietary and lifestyle changes take place over time. It is a process of replacing bad habits with good habits. However, the need for hormonal supplementation still exists. It is important to keep in mind that the market for "natural" hormone products is a multibillion dollar market, and without strict quality controls, there is the potential for supplements to be considered "safe" when in actuality, the long term affects could be devastating. Be cautious of sensational claims made for over-the-counter products. Make sure to consult with a qualified professional health care provider to insure the individual needs are being met. "All natural" does not mean "all safe". Preliminary studies do not justify long term use. When dealing with the endocrine system, the complexity and internal balances are delicate, and random supplementing with over-the-counter "miracle pills" could lead to more serious problems in the future. This is not to say that one should not seek out the most natural forms of treatment. Decisions and actions should be predicated on adequate research.

The information presented has been designed to provide education and awareness for the growing force of individuals searching for the best natural forms of treatment when dealing with PMS (premenstrual syndrome), peri-menopause, pre-menopause and menopause. Because the endocrine system is quite volatile, sometimes the only way to know what is best is purely by trial and error. Although trial and error is less than scientific, each person is unique and how one specific product will perform can vary greatly between individuals.

The prescription is to take control of individual health and wellness. Learn to identify the signs the body is giving through the symptoms being experienced. Understand it is completely possible to integrate allopathic and naturopathic practices when it comes to achieving optimal health. The integration can only result in better health care for everyone.

Become educated and informed when dealing with "natural" products. The regulations governing "supplements" are far different than those governing prescriptions.

Balance needs to first come from nature. The food one eats, the air one breathes, the water one drinks and the lifestyle one lives are all controlled individually and are personal choices.

Remember you are in charge and make your decisions based on the best information available.

Life choices must be informed choices!

Index

L

M

N

O

P